DELMAR'S MATH REVIEW *FOR* HEALTH CARE PROFESSIONALS

THE BASICS OF FRACTIONS

✓ W9-AGK-991

Roger W. Ellsbury

**Associate Professor
Goodwin College
East Hartford, CT**

&

**Evening Supervisor
Stone Academy
Waterbury, CT**

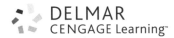

DELMAR
CENGAGE Learning™

Australia • Brazil • Japan • Korea • Mexico • Singapore • Spain • United Kingdom • United States

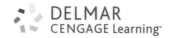
DELMAR
CENGAGE Learning™

Delmar's Math Review for Health Care Professionals: The Basics of Fractions
Roger W. Ellsbury

Vice President, Editorial: Dave Garza

Director of Learning Solutions: Matthew Kane

Executive Editor: Stephen Helba

Senior Acquisitions Editor: Maureen Rosener

Managing Editor: Marah Bellegarde

Editorial Assistant: Samantha Miller

Vice President, Career and Professional
Marketing: Jennifer Baker

Marketing Director: Wendy E. Mapstone

Senior Marketing Manager: Michele McTighe

Marketing Coordinator: Scott A. Chrysler

Senior Production Director: Wendy A. Troeger

Production Manager: Andrew Crouth

Content Project Management: PreMediaGlobal

Compositor: PreMediaGlobal

For product information and technology assistance, contact us at
Cengage Learning Customer & Sales Support, 1-800-354-9706

For permission to use material from this text or product,
submit all requests online at **www.cengage.com/permissions**.
Further permissions questions can be e-mailed to
permissionrequest@cengage.com

Library of Congress Control Number: 2011937711

ISBN-13: 978-1-4390-5835-0

ISBN-10: 1-4390-5835-0

Delmar
5 Maxwell Drive
Clifton Park, NY 12065-2919
USA

Cengage Learning is a leading provider of customized learning solutions with office locations around the globe, including Singapore, the United Kingdom, Australia, Mexico, Brazil, and Japan. Locate your local office at: **international.cengage.com/region**

Cengage Learning products are represented in Canada by
Nelson Education, Ltd.

To learn more about Delmar, visit **www.cengage.com/delmar**

Purchase any of our products at your local college store or at our preferred online store **www.cengagebrain.com**

Printed in the United States of America
1 2 3 4 5 6 7 15 14 13 12 11

TABLE OF CONTENTS

DELMAR'S MATH REVIEW SERIES FOR HEALTH CARE PROFESSIONALS

This series is designed to assist students who are studying to become health care professionals, those just entering the health care field, and practicing health care professionals who need to review mathematical concepts. This series assumes that the reader has basic arithmetic skills, particularly a basic understanding of fraction concepts. This series is an ideal companion to a dosage calculation book.

This series is designed as small modules of topic-specific math content. This modular design allows readers the flexibility to choose the areas they want to study. In addition, the books in the series can be used in a classroom or an online class setting, where an instructor presents the material and students practice the concepts presented, or can be used as supplemental material for readers who want to review the concepts on their own. The explanations and examples are clear enough for readers to follow independently.

The series is designed to enhance the reader's learning experience. The instructional sections are presented in a clear and straightforward manner without distracting graphics or colors. The emphasis is on a basic presentation of the concepts with numerous examples and explanations to illustrate their various applications. The reader has many opportunities to practice the concepts, and answers and explanations to the questions are included so that the reader can immediately check an answer and remediate as necessary.

Series Organization:

This four-book module series includes:

Basics of Decimals/ISBN: 1-4390-5837-7

Basics of Fractions/ISBN: 1-4390-5835-0

Basics of Percents/ISBN: 1-4390-5836-9

Basics of Rate, Ratio, and Proportion/ISBN: 1-4390-5838-5

Book Features

Each book contains the following features designed to provide students with straightforward explanations of concepts, examples, practice, and testing situations to check their comprehension of content.

- Each book is organized into small *Sections* to enhance the reading experience.

- *Learning Objectives* found at the beginning of each section focus the reader on the concepts to be covered.

- Multiple *Examples* afford readers several opportunities to gain an understanding of the content.

- *Exercises,* found after each concept presentation, allow readers to check their comprehension before moving on to new content.

- A *Section Test* is included at the end of each section. Here students assess their understanding of the concepts they studied.

- *Answers* with detailed explanations for all Exercises, all Review Exercises, and the Section Test are included at the end of each section, allowing readers to check their work and remediate as necessary.

- A *Summary* contains all of the important information presented in the book. Readers can review the Summary before taking the Cumulative Test. Readers also will find the Summary to be an invaluable reference for future use.

- A *Cumulative Test* allows students to assess their knowledge of all concepts presented in the book. The *Answers* are provided immediately after the test.

Roger Ellsbury is a full-time Associate Professor at Goodwin College in East Hartford, Connecticut, where he has been teaching math, English, and computer courses for seven years. His extensive background as an educator included 25 years of public school teaching, after which time he became Senior Facilitator for the Academy of Learning in Waterbury, Connecticut, teaching end-user software to adults.

Continuing his career as an educator, he accepted a position as instructor of Integrated Computer Technology at Stone Academy in Waterbury, where he taught Mathematics for Science and Technology along with various courses in computer technology. Later he taught Medical Terminology, Medical Law and Ethics, Professional Development, Business Communications, English Fundamentals, and Communication Skills for Healthcare Professionals. While at Stone Academy, he was promoted to and currently holds the position of Evening Supervisor. In this position, he is responsible for the staff, faculty, and students in the evening programs. He has also conducted in-service training sessions in computer software for the staff and faculty.

After receiving a Bachelor of Arts and a Master of Arts degrees at the University of Connecticut, Roger continued his studies at Saint Joseph College in Connecticut. He earned a Certificate of Advanced Graduate Study (CAGS) in special education. In the field of computer technology, he has earned A+, Network+, and Microsoft Office User Specialist (Master Level) certifications. He has also received a Diploma from the Academy of Learning in Computer Software Applications.

ACKNOWLEDGMENTS

I would like to thank Goodwin College for its continuing support with this project.

I also would like to thank all the people at Delmar/Cengage Learning who have had a hand in this project, especially Maureen Rosener whose vision and understanding has helped turn my idea into reality. Her guidance and suggestions have been invaluable.

I would especially like to thank my wife, Linda, for her support, tolerance, and patience. Her advice based on years of experience in education and her excellent proofreading abilities have made this project even better.

Michele Bach, MS
Mathematics Professor
Kansas City, Kansas Community College
Kansas City, KS

Patricia Sunderhaus, EdD(c), MSN, RN
Practical Nursing Coordinator
Brown Mackie College
Cincinnati, OH

Margie Washnok, ARPN, MS, DNP
Professor
Presentation College
Aberdeen, SD

Fraction Concepts

OBJECTIVES

Upon completion of this section, you should be able to:

1) Explain basic fraction concepts.

2) Reduce a fraction to its lowest terms.

3) Change a mixed number to an improper fraction.

4) Change a whole number to an improper fraction.

5) Change an improper fraction to a whole number or a mixed number.

WHAT IS A FRACTION?

A **fraction** is a method of division and is used to indicate a part of a whole. A fraction consists of an upper number called the **numerator** and a lower number called the **denominator**. They are separated by a horizontal line.

For the fraction $\frac{3}{4}$, the denominator 4 indicates that one whole unit is divided into 4 parts. The numerator 3 indicates that this fraction consists of three of the 4 parts.

Example 1

1a) *What does the fraction $\frac{4}{5}$ mean?*

The denominator 5 means that one whole unit is divided into 5 parts. The numerator 4 means that this fraction has 4 of these parts.

1b) *What does the fraction $\frac{2}{3}$ mean?*

The denominator 3 means that one whole unit is divided into 3 parts. The numerator 2 means that this fraction has 2 of these parts.

1c) *What does the fraction $\frac{5}{8}$ mean?*

The denominator 8 means that one whole unit is divided into 8 parts. The numerator 5 means that this fraction has 5 of these parts.

REDUCING A FRACTION TO ITS LOWEST TERMS

If a number can divide evenly into both the numerator and the denominator of a fraction without having a remainder, then the fraction can be reduced by that number. If there is more than one number that can reduce a fraction, use the larger number to save steps.

If there is no number that can divide evenly into both the numerator and the denominator, then the fraction cannot be reduced. If a fraction cannot be reduced, the fraction is in its **lowest terms**. A final answer should have a fraction reduced to its lowest terms.

Example 2

2a) *What number can divide evenly into the numerator and denominator of $\frac{2}{4}$?*

The number 2 can divide evenly into the numerator 2 and the denominator 4: $\frac{2 \div 2}{4 \div 2} = \frac{1}{2}$. This fraction cannot be reduced any further.

2b) *What number can divide evenly into the numerator and denominator of $\frac{6}{9}$?*

The number 3 can divide evenly into the numerator 6 and the denominator 9: $\frac{6 \div 3}{9 \div 3} = \frac{2}{3}$. This fraction cannot be reduced any further.

2c) *What number can divide evenly into the numerator and denominator of $\frac{4}{8}$?*

Both the numbers 2 and 4 can divide evenly into the numerator 4 and the denominator 8. If we use the number 2, then $\frac{4 \div 2}{8 \div 2} = \frac{2}{4}$. This fraction still can be reduced by 2. If we use the number 4, then $\frac{4 \div 4}{8 \div 4} = \frac{1}{2}$. This fraction cannot be reduced any further.

2d) *What number can divide evenly into the numerator and denominator of $\frac{6}{12}$?*

The numbers 2, 3, and 6 can divide evenly into the numerator 6 and the denominator 12. If we use the number 2, then $\frac{6 \div 2}{12 \div 2} = \frac{3}{6}$. This fraction can still be reduced by 3. If we use the number 3, then $\frac{6 \div 3}{12 \div 3} = \frac{2}{4}$. This fraction can still be reduced by 2. If we use the number 6, then $\frac{6 \div 6}{12 \div 6} = \frac{1}{2}$. This fraction cannot be reduced any further.

Note: If there is more than one number that can reduce a fraction, use the larger number to save steps.

EXERCISES IN REDUCING FRACTIONS

(Answers are on page 14.)

Reduce these fractions to their lowest terms.

1) $\dfrac{5}{10}$

2) $\dfrac{4}{16}$

3) $\dfrac{6}{8}$

4) $\dfrac{3}{9}$

5) $\dfrac{30}{50}$

6) $\dfrac{6}{18}$

7) $\dfrac{7}{21}$

8) $\dfrac{12}{18}$

9) $\dfrac{25}{40}$

10) $\dfrac{21}{24}$

11) $\dfrac{9}{81}$

12) $\dfrac{44}{99}$

13) $\dfrac{8}{32}$

14) $\dfrac{20}{24}$

15) $\dfrac{16}{32}$

16) $\dfrac{24}{48}$

17) $\dfrac{20}{80}$

18) $\dfrac{21}{35}$

FORMS OF A FRACTION

> There are three forms of a fraction: proper fraction, improper fraction, and mixed number.
>
> A **proper fraction** has a denominator that is larger than the numerator. $\frac{3}{5}$ is an example of a proper fraction.
>
> An **improper fraction** has a numerator that is equal to or larger than the denominator. $\frac{5}{3}$ and $\frac{4}{4}$ are examples of improper fractions. When the numerator and denominator are equal, then the fraction can be reduced to 1.
>
> A **mixed number** is a combination of a whole number and a fraction. $1\frac{2}{3}$ is an example of a mixed number.

Example 3

Identify the fraction as a proper fraction, an improper fraction, or a mixed number.

3a) $\frac{7}{12}$ This is a proper fraction because the denominator is larger than the numerator. If a triangle were drawn around the fraction with the horizontal side nearest the larger number, it would look like Figure 1-1.

Figure 1-1

3b) $\frac{9}{5}$ This is an improper fraction because the numerator is larger than the denominator. If a triangle were drawn around the fraction with the horizontal side nearest the larger number, it would look like Figure 1-2.

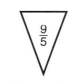

Figure 1-2

3c) $\frac{8}{8}$ This is an improper fraction because the numerator is equal to the denominator. This fraction can be reduced to 1 by dividing the numerator and denominator by 8.

3d) $5\frac{3}{4}$ This is a mixed number because it is a combination of a whole number and a fraction. 5 is the whole number and $\frac{3}{4}$ is the fraction.

EXERCISES IN IDENTIFYING THE FORMS OF A FRACTION

(Answers are on page 15.)

Identify the fraction as a proper fraction, an improper fraction, or a mixed number.

1) $\frac{5}{9}$

2) $\frac{13}{7}$

3) $9\frac{2}{7}$

4) $\frac{14}{14}$

5) $1\frac{3}{4}$

6) $\frac{3}{16}$

7) $\frac{9}{8}$

8) $4\frac{5}{8}$

9) $\frac{5}{21}$

10) $2\frac{13}{16}$

11) $\frac{20}{17}$

12) $\frac{9}{9}$

CHANGING AN IMPROPER FRACTION TO A WHOLE NUMBER OR A MIXED NUMBER

To change an improper fraction to a whole number or a mixed number, follow these steps.

Step 1:   Divide the denominator into the numerator. The answer (without the remainder) is the whole-number part of the mixed number.

Step 2:   Write the remainder part of the answer as the numerator with the divisor of the fraction as the denominator. If there is no remainder, then the answer is just a whole number.

Step 3:   Reduce the fraction if possible.

Note: If there is no remainder, then the answer is a whole number, not a mixed number.

To turn $\frac{5}{3}$ into a mixed number, divide 3 into 5.

$$3)\overline{5} \quad \frac{1}{} \quad \frac{3}{2}$$

It goes in 1 time with a remainder of 2. The whole number in the mixed number is 1, the numerator of the fraction is 2, and the denominator of the fraction is 3.

Thus, $\frac{5}{3}$ as a mixed number is $1\frac{2}{3}$

Example 4

Change these fractions into whole numbers or mixed numbers.

4a) $\frac{17}{5}$ 5 divides into 17 a total of 3 times with a remainder of 2. The mixed number is $3\frac{2}{5}$

$$5)\overline{17} \quad \frac{3}{} \quad \frac{15}{2}$$

4b) $\frac{24}{9}$ 9 divides into 24 a total of 2 times with a remainder of 6. The mixed number is $2\frac{6}{9}$ which reduces to $2\frac{2}{3}$

$$9)\overline{24} \quad \frac{2}{} \quad \frac{18}{6}$$

4c) $\frac{21}{7}$ 7 divides into 21 a total of 3 times with no remainder. The answer is the whole number 3 with no fraction.

$$7)\overline{21} \quad \frac{3}{} \quad \frac{21}{0}$$

EXERCISES IN CHANGING IMPROPER FRACTIONS
TO WHOLE NUMBERS OR MIXED NUMBERS

(Answers are on page 15.)

Change these improper fractions to whole or mixed numbers. Reduce if possible.

1) $\frac{13}{7}$ 2) $\frac{34}{4}$ 3) $\frac{42}{5}$

4) $\frac{28}{14}$ 5) $\frac{20}{8}$ 6) $\frac{48}{10}$

7) $\frac{33}{9}$ 8) $\frac{14}{6}$ 9) $\frac{45}{6}$

10) $\frac{24}{4}$ 11) $\frac{96}{9}$ 12) $\frac{50}{8}$

CHANGING A WHOLE NUMBER TO AN IMPROPER FRACTION

> To change a whole number to an improper fraction, place the whole number in the numerator and use a denominator of 1.
>
> To change 6 to an improper fraction, place 6 in the numerator and use a denominator of 1. Thus, $6 = \frac{6}{1}$

Example 5

Change these whole numbers into improper fractions.

5a) 3   Place 3 in the numerator over a denominator of 1. Thus, $3 = \frac{3}{1}$

5b) 16   Place 16 in the numerator over a denominator of 1. Thus, $16 = \frac{16}{1}$

5c) 1   Place 1 in the numerator over a denominator of 1. Thus, $1 = \frac{1}{1}$

CHANGING A MIXED NUMBER TO AN IMPROPER FRACTION

To change a mixed number to an improper fraction, follow these steps:

Step 1: Multiply the denominator times the whole-number part of the mixed number.

Step 2: Add the answer of Step 1 to the numerator of the mixed number.

Step 3: Place this total over the same denominator of the mixed number.

To change $2\frac{3}{4}$ to an improper fraction, multiply the denominator 4 times the whole number 2 to get 8. Next, add 8 to the numerator 3 to get a total of 11. Place 11 in the numerator with the original denominator of 4. Thus, $2\frac{3}{4} = \frac{11}{4}$

Example 6

Change these mixed numbers into improper fractions.

6a) $3\frac{1}{2}$ Multiply 2 times 3 and add 1 to get 7. Thus, $3\frac{1}{2} = \frac{7}{2}$

6b) $2\frac{5}{8}$ Multiply 8 times 2 and add 5 to get 21. Thus, $2\frac{5}{8} = \frac{21}{8}$

6c) $8\frac{3}{4}$ Multiply 4 times 8 and add 3 to get 35. Thus, $8\frac{3}{4} = \frac{35}{4}$

6d) $2\frac{5}{12}$ Multiply 12 times 2 and add 5 to get 29. Thus, $2\frac{5}{12} = \frac{29}{12}$

EXERCISES IN CHANGING WHOLE NUMBERS AND MIXED NUMBERS TO IMPROPER FRACTIONS

(Answers are on pages 15–16.)

Change these whole numbers and mixed numbers into improper fractions.

1) 2

2) $5\frac{3}{4}$

3) $2\frac{2}{3}$

4) $6\frac{2}{5}$

5) $10\frac{3}{8}$

6) 9

7) $3\frac{7}{9}$

8) $2\frac{5}{12}$

9) $3\frac{5}{6}$

10) $1\frac{4}{5}$

11) 100

12) $6\frac{7}{8}$

SECTION TEST: FRACTION CONCEPTS

(*The answers are on page 16.*)

1)   In the fraction $\frac{2}{3}$, what number is the denominator?

2)   In the fraction $\frac{2}{3}$, what number is the numerator?

3)   In the fraction $\frac{2}{3}$, what does the 3 mean?

4)   In the fraction $\frac{2}{3}$, what does the 2 mean?

Identify each of the following as a proper fraction, improper fraction, or mixed number.

5) $\frac{9}{5}$ 6) $\frac{3}{4}$ 7) $3\frac{1}{3}$ 8) $\frac{7}{4}$

Reduce the following fractions to their lowest terms.

9) $\frac{4}{8}$ 10) $\frac{3}{9}$ 11) $\frac{15}{20}$ 12) $\frac{12}{18}$

13) $\frac{8}{12}$ 14) $\frac{25}{40}$ 15) $\frac{25}{75}$ 16) $\frac{12}{16}$

Change these improper fractions to either whole numbers or mixed numbers.

17) $\frac{13}{8}$ 18) $\frac{9}{5}$ 19) $\frac{12}{4}$ 20) $\frac{17}{2}$

21) $\frac{4}{3}$ 22) $\frac{15}{4}$ 23) $\frac{16}{8}$ 24) $\frac{36}{12}$

Change these whole numbers or mixed numbers into improper fractions.

25) $1\frac{1}{8}$ 26) $2\frac{3}{4}$ 27) $5\frac{5}{8}$ 28) 6

29) $3\frac{4}{5}$ 30) 15   31) $3\frac{2}{7}$ 32) $7\frac{8}{9}$

ANSWERS TO EXERCISES IN REDUCING FRACTIONS

(*Exercises are on page 4.*)

1) Divide the numerator and denominator by 5. Thus, $\frac{5}{10} = \frac{1}{2}$

2) Divide the numerator and denominator by 4. Thus, $\frac{4}{16} = \frac{1}{4}$

3) Divide the numerator and denominator by 2. Thus, $\frac{6}{8} = \frac{3}{4}$

4) Divide the numerator and denominator by 3. Thus, $\frac{3}{9} = \frac{1}{3}$

5) Divide the numerator and denominator by 10. Thus, $\frac{30}{50} = \frac{3}{5}$

6) Divide the numerator and denominator by 6. Thus, $\frac{6}{18} = \frac{1}{3}$

7) Divide the numerator and denominator by 7. Thus, $\frac{7}{21} = \frac{1}{3}$

8) Divide the numerator and denominator by 6. Thus, $\frac{12}{18} = \frac{2}{3}$

9) Divide the numerator and denominator by 5. Thus, $\frac{25}{40} = \frac{5}{8}$

10) Divide the numerator and denominator by 3. Thus, $\frac{21}{24} = \frac{7}{8}$

11) Divide the numerator and denominator by 9. Thus, $\frac{9}{81} = \frac{1}{9}$

12) Divide the numerator and denominator by 11. Thus, $\frac{44}{99} = \frac{4}{9}$

13) Divide the numerator and denominator by 8. Thus, $\frac{8}{32} = \frac{1}{4}$

14) Divide the numerator and denominator by 4. Thus, $\frac{20}{24} = \frac{5}{6}$

15) Divide the numerator and denominator by 16. Thus, $\frac{16}{32} = \frac{1}{2}$

16) Divide the numerator and denominator by 24. Thus, $\frac{24}{48} = \frac{1}{2}$

17) Divide the numerator and denominator by 20. Thus, $\frac{20}{80} = \frac{1}{4}$

18) Divide the numerator and denominator by 7. Thus, $\frac{21}{35} = \frac{3}{5}$

ANSWERS TO EXERCISES IN IDENTIFYING THE FORMS OF A FRACTION

(*Exercises are on page 6.*)

1) $\frac{5}{9}$ is a proper fraction.

2) $\frac{13}{7}$ is an improper fraction.

3) $9\frac{2}{7}$ is a mixed number.

4) $\frac{14}{14}$ is an improper fraction.

5) $1\frac{3}{4}$ is a mixed number.

6) $\frac{3}{16}$ is a proper fraction.

7) $\frac{9}{8}$ is an improper fraction.

8) $4\frac{5}{8}$ is a mixed number.

9) $\frac{5}{21}$ is a proper fraction.

10) $2\frac{13}{16}$ is a mixed number.

11) $\frac{20}{17}$ is an improper fraction.

12) $\frac{9}{9}$ is an improper fraction.

ANSWERS TO EXERCISES IN CHANGING IMPROPER FRACTIONS TO WHOLE NUMBERS OR MIXED NUMBERS

(*Exercises are on page 8.*)

1) $\frac{13}{7} = 1\frac{6}{7}$

2) $\frac{34}{4} = 8\frac{2}{4} = 8\frac{1}{2}$

3) $\frac{42}{5} = 8\frac{2}{5}$

4) $\frac{28}{14} = 2$

5) $\frac{20}{8} = 2\frac{4}{8} = 2\frac{1}{2}$

6) $\frac{48}{10} = 4\frac{8}{10} = 4\frac{4}{5}$

7) $\frac{33}{9} = 3\frac{6}{9} = 3\frac{2}{3}$

8) $\frac{14}{6} = 2\frac{2}{6} = 2\frac{1}{3}$

9) $\frac{45}{6} = 7\frac{3}{6} = 7\frac{1}{2}$

10) $\frac{24}{4} = 6$

11) $\frac{96}{9} = 10\frac{6}{9} = 10\frac{2}{3}$

12) $\frac{50}{8} = 6\frac{2}{8} = 6\frac{1}{4}$

ANSWERS TO EXERCISES IN CHANGING WHOLE NUMBERS AND MIXED NUMBERS TO IMPROPER FRACTIONS

(*Exercises are on page 11.*)

1) $2 = \frac{2}{1}$

2) $5\frac{3}{4} = \frac{23}{4}$

3) $2\frac{2}{3} = \frac{8}{3}$

4) $6\frac{2}{5} = \frac{32}{5}$

5) $10\frac{3}{8} = \frac{83}{8}$

6) $9 = \frac{9}{1}$

7) $3\frac{7}{9} = \frac{34}{9}$

8) $2\frac{5}{12} = \frac{29}{12}$

9) $3\frac{5}{6} = \frac{23}{6}$

10) $1\frac{4}{5} = \frac{9}{5}$

11) $100 = \frac{100}{1}$

12) $6\frac{7}{8} = \frac{55}{8}$

ANSWERS TO SECTION TEST: FRACTION CONCEPTS
(*Section Test is on pages 12–13.*)

1) In the fraction $\frac{2}{3}$, 3 is the denominator.

2) In the fraction $\frac{2}{3}$, 2 is the numerator

3) In the fraction $\frac{2}{3}$, one whole is divided into 3 parts.

4) In the fraction $\frac{2}{3}$, 2 indicates that this fraction has 2 of the 3 parts.

5) $\frac{9}{5}$ is an improper fraction.

6) $\frac{3}{4}$ is a proper fraction.

7) $3\frac{1}{3}$ is a mixed number.

8) $\frac{7}{4}$ is an improper fraction.

9) $\frac{4}{8} = \frac{1}{2}$

10) $\frac{3}{9} = \frac{1}{3}$

11) $\frac{15}{20} = \frac{3}{4}$

12) $\frac{12}{18} = \frac{2}{3}$

13) $\frac{8}{12} = \frac{2}{3}$

14) $\frac{25}{40} = \frac{5}{8}$

15) $\frac{25}{75} = \frac{1}{3}$

16) $\frac{12}{16} = \frac{3}{4}$

17) $\frac{13}{8} = 1\frac{5}{8}$

18) $\frac{9}{5} = 1\frac{4}{5}$

19) $\frac{12}{4} = 3$

20) $\frac{17}{2} = 8\frac{1}{2}$

21) $\frac{4}{3} = 1\frac{1}{3}$

22) $\frac{15}{4} = 3\frac{3}{4}$

23) $\frac{16}{8} = 2$

24) $\frac{36}{12} = 3$

25) $1\frac{1}{8} = \frac{9}{8}$

26) $2\frac{3}{4} = \frac{11}{4}$

27) $5\frac{5}{8} = \frac{45}{8}$

28) $6 = \frac{6}{1}$

29) $3\frac{4}{5} = \frac{19}{5}$

30) $15 = \frac{15}{1}$

31) $3\frac{2}{7} = \frac{23}{7}$

32) $7\frac{8}{9} = \frac{71}{9}$

Addition of Fractions

OBJECTIVES

Upon completion of this section, you should be able to:

1) Add fractions with like denominators.

2) Find the least common multiple and lowest common denominator of a group of fractions.

3) Raise a fraction to higher terms.

4) Add fractions with unlike denominators.

5) Add mixed numbers.

6) Solve application problems using fractions.

ADDING FRACTIONS WITH LIKE DENOMINATORS

To add fractions with like denominators, add the numerators and use the same denominator. For example, 2 and 3 equal 5.

$$\frac{2}{7} + \frac{3}{7} = \frac{5}{7}$$

Frequently, when adding fractions, the answer may have to be changed to a mixed number and reduced.

Example 1

1a) *Add* $\frac{4}{17} + \frac{6}{17}$

Add the numerators 4 and 6 to get 10. Place 10 in the numerator with 17 as the denominator. Thus, $\frac{4}{17} + \frac{6}{17} = \frac{10}{17}$

1b) *Add* $\frac{8}{23} + \frac{11}{23}$

Add the numerators 8 and 11 to get 19. Place 19 in the numerator with 23 as the denominator. Thus, $\frac{8}{23} + \frac{11}{23} = \frac{19}{23}$

Example 2

2a) *Add* $\frac{8}{20} + \frac{4}{20}$

Add the numerators 8 and 4 to get 12. Place 12 in the numerator with 20 as the denominator. Reduce the answer.

Thus, $\frac{8}{20} + \frac{4}{20} = \frac{12}{20} = \frac{3}{5}$

2b) *Add* $\frac{5}{12} + \frac{3}{12}$

Add the numerators 5 and 3 to get 8. Place 8 in the numerator with 12 as the denominator. Reduce the answer.

Thus, $\frac{5}{12} + \frac{3}{12} = \frac{8}{12} = \frac{2}{3}$

Example 3

3a) *Add* $\frac{5}{9} + \frac{8}{9}$

Add the numerators 5 and 8 to get 13. Place 13 in the numerator with 9 as the denominator. Convert the answer to a mixed number.

Thus, $\frac{5}{9} + \frac{8}{9} = \frac{13}{9} = 1\frac{4}{9}$

3b) *Add* $\frac{3}{4} + \frac{3}{4}$

Add the numerators 3 and 3 to get 6. Place 6 in the numerator with 4 as the denominator. Convert the answer to a mixed number and reduce.

Thus, $\frac{3}{4} + \frac{3}{4} = \frac{6}{4} = 1\frac{2}{4} = 1\frac{1}{2}$

3c) *Add* $\frac{9}{16} + \frac{7}{16}$

Add the numerators 9 and 7 to get 16. Place 16 in the numerator with 16 as the denominator. Convert the answer to a whole number.

Thus, $\frac{9}{16} + \frac{7}{16} = \frac{16}{16} = 1$

EXERCISES IN ADDING FRACTIONS WITH LIKE DENOMINATORS

(Answers are on page 43.)

Add these fractions. If the answer is an improper fraction, convert it to a mixed number. Reduce if possible.

1) $\frac{4}{11} + \frac{5}{11}$

2) $\frac{7}{25} + \frac{12}{25}$

3) $\frac{15}{47} + \frac{15}{47}$

4) $\frac{3}{5} + \frac{2}{5}$

5) $\frac{4}{13} + \frac{6}{13}$

6) $\frac{4}{9} + \frac{7}{9}$

7) $\dfrac{2}{15} + \dfrac{4}{15} + \dfrac{1}{15}$

8) $\dfrac{7}{9} + \dfrac{2}{9} + \dfrac{5}{9}$

9) $\dfrac{5}{8} + \dfrac{7}{8} + \dfrac{3}{8} + \dfrac{1}{8}$

10) $\dfrac{9}{10} + \dfrac{9}{10}$

11) $\dfrac{3}{8} + \dfrac{7}{8}$

12) $\dfrac{5}{12} + \dfrac{11}{12}$

FINDING THE LEAST COMMON MULTIPLE OF A SET OF NUMBERS

The **common multiples** of a set of numbers are multiples that can be divided evenly by all of the numbers in the set.

Consider the set of 2 and 3. Their multiples are:
Multiples of 3: 3, <u>6</u>, 9, <u>12</u>, 15, <u>18</u>, 21 ...
Multiples of 2: 2, 4, <u>6</u>, 8, 10, <u>12</u>, 14, 16, <u>18</u>, 20 ...

The numbers that 2 and 3 share in common from this list are 6, 12, and 18. The lowest number is 6. This is called the least common multiple.

The **least common multiple** of a set of numbers is the lowest multiple into which all of the numbers in the set can divide evenly.

Use the least common multiple as the lowest common denominator for a group of fractions. The **lowest common denominator** (**LCD**) is the smallest number that can be divided evenly by all of the denominators in the group of fractions.

Example 4

4a) *What is the least common multiple of 3 and 4?*

First write the multiples of each number, looking for the lowest number they have in common. List a few multiples of the larger number in the set and then list the multiples of the smaller number.

Multiples of 4: 4, 8, <u>12</u>, 16, 20, <u>24</u>, 28 ...

Multiples of 3: 3, 6, 9, <u>12</u>, 15, 18, 21, <u>24</u>, 27 ...

The least common multiple of 3 and 4 is 12. Note that 24 is also a common multiple, but it is not the **lowest** one.

4b) *What is the least common multiple of 2 and 5?*

The multiples of 5: 5, <u>10</u>, 15 ...

The multiples of 2: 2, 4, 6, 8, <u>10</u>, 12, 14 ...

The least common multiple of 2 and 5 is 10.

4c) *What is the least common multiple of 3, 5, and 6?*

The multiples of 6: 6, 12, 18, 24, <u>30</u>, 36 ...

The multiples of 5: 5, 10, 15, 20, 25, <u>30</u>, 35 ...

The multiples of 3: 3, 6, 9, 12, 15, 18, 21, 24, 27, <u>30</u>, 33 ...

The least common multiple of 3, 5, and 6 is 30.

EXERCISES IN FINDING THE LEAST COMMON MULTIPLE OF A SET OF NUMBERS

(Answers are on page 43.)

1)   *What is the least common multiple of 4 and 5?*

2)   *What is the least common multiple of 6 and 8?*

3)   *What is the least common multiple of 2, 3, and 5?*

RAISING A FRACTION TO A HIGHER TERM

> If a number is multiplied by both the numerator and the denominator, the fraction is raised to a higher term. The amount the fraction represents does not change. Think of this as the opposite of reducing a fraction.
>
> To raise a fraction to a higher term, multiply the numerator and the denominator by the same number.

Example 5

5a) *Raise $\frac{3}{5}$ to $\frac{}{20}$*

Divide 5 into 20 to get 4. This means 5 was multiplied by 4 to get 20. The numerator must also be multiplied by 4 to keep the fraction equivalent to the original. 3 times $4 = 12$. Thus, $\frac{3 \times 4}{5 \times 4} = \frac{12}{20}$

5b) *Raise $\frac{1}{2}$ to $\frac{}{10}$*

Divide 2 into 10 to get 5. This means 2 was multiplied by 5 to get 10. The numerator must also be multiplied by 5 to keep the fraction equivalent to the original. 1 times $5 = 5$. Thus, $\frac{1 \times 5}{2 \times 5} = \frac{5}{10}$

5c) *Raise $\frac{2}{3}$ to $\frac{}{21}$*

Divide 3 into 21 to get 7. This means 3 was multiplied by 7 to get 21. The numerator must also be multiplied by 7 to keep the fraction equivalent to the original. 2 times $7 = 14$. Thus, $\frac{2 \times 7}{3 \times 7} = \frac{14}{21}$

EXERCISES IN RAISING A FRACTION TO A HIGHER TERM

(Answers are on page 44.)

Raise each fraction to its equivalent higher term by supplying the missing numerator.

1) $\dfrac{1}{2} = \dfrac{}{6}$

2) $\dfrac{2}{3} = \dfrac{}{15}$

3) $\dfrac{3}{4} = \dfrac{}{24}$

4) $\dfrac{2}{5} = \dfrac{}{35}$

5) $\dfrac{1}{6} = \dfrac{}{18}$

6) $\dfrac{4}{7} = \dfrac{}{21}$

7) $\dfrac{3}{10} = \dfrac{}{70}$

8) $\dfrac{7}{12} = \dfrac{}{48}$

9) $\dfrac{1}{2} = \dfrac{}{16}$

ADDING FRACTIONS WITH UNLIKE DENOMINATORS

> To add fractions with unlike denominators, follow these steps.
>
> Step 1: Find the lowest common denominator for the fractions to be added.
>
> Step 2: Change one or more of the fractions so the fractions all have the same denominators.
>
> Step 3: Add the fractions.
>
> Step 4: If necessary, change the answer to a mixed number and reduce when possible.

Example 6

6a) *Add* $\frac{1}{2} + \frac{1}{4}$

$$\frac{1}{2} = \frac{1 \times 2}{2 \times 2} = \frac{2}{4}$$
$$+\frac{1}{4} \qquad = \frac{1}{4}$$
$$\overline{\qquad \frac{3}{4}}$$

The LCD for these fractions is 4. Change $\frac{1}{2}$ to $\frac{2}{4}$. The fraction $\frac{1}{4}$ need not be changed. Add the numerators: $2 + 1 = 3$. The answer is $\frac{3}{4}$. This is a proper fraction and need not be reduced.

Thus, $\frac{1}{2} + \frac{1}{4} = \frac{3}{4}$

6b) *Add* $\frac{2}{3} + \frac{3}{4}$

$$\frac{2}{3} = \frac{2 \times 4}{3 \times 4} = \frac{8}{12}$$
$$+\frac{3}{4} = \frac{3 \times 3}{4 \times 3} = \frac{9}{12}$$
$$\overline{\qquad \frac{17}{12} = 1\frac{5}{12}}$$

The LCD for these fractions is 12. Change $\frac{2}{3}$ to $\frac{8}{12}$, and change $\frac{3}{4}$ to $\frac{9}{12}$. Add the numerators. $8 + 9 = 17$. The answer is $\frac{17}{12}$. Turn this improper fraction into a mixed number.

Thus, $\frac{2}{3} + \frac{3}{4} = 1\frac{5}{12}$

6c) *Add* $\frac{5}{6} + \frac{2}{3}$

$$\frac{5}{6} \qquad = \frac{5}{6}$$
$$+\frac{2}{3} = \frac{2 \times 2}{3 \times 2} = \frac{4}{6}$$
$$\overline{\qquad\qquad\qquad} \\ \frac{9}{6} = 1\frac{3}{6} = 1\frac{1}{2}$$

The LCD for these fractions is 6. Change $\frac{2}{3}$ to $\frac{4}{6}$. $\frac{5}{6}$ need not be changed. Add the numerators. $5 + 4 = 9$. The answer is $\frac{9}{6}$. Turn this improper fraction into a mixed number and then reduce.

Thus, $\frac{5}{6} + \frac{2}{3} = 1\frac{1}{2}$

6d) *Add* $\frac{4}{5} + \frac{3}{4}$

$$\frac{4}{5} = \frac{4 \times 4}{5 \times 4} = \frac{16}{20}$$
$$+\frac{3}{4} = \frac{3 \times 5}{4 \times 5} = \frac{15}{20}$$
$$\overline{\qquad\qquad\qquad} \\ \frac{31}{20} = 1\frac{11}{20}$$

The LCD for these fractions is 20. Change $\frac{4}{5}$ to $\frac{16}{20}$, and $\frac{3}{4}$ to $\frac{15}{20}$. Add the numerators: $16 + 15 = 31$. The answer is $\frac{31}{20}$. Turn this improper fraction into a mixed number.

Thus, $\frac{4}{5} + \frac{3}{4} = 1\frac{11}{20}$

6e) *Add* $\frac{5}{6} + \frac{2}{3} + \frac{3}{4}$

$$\frac{5}{6} = \frac{5 \times 2}{6 \times 2} = \frac{10}{12}$$
$$\frac{2}{3} = \frac{2 \times 4}{3 \times 4} = \frac{8}{12}$$
$$+\frac{3}{4} = \frac{3 \times 3}{4 \times 3} = \frac{9}{12}$$
$$\overline{\qquad\qquad\qquad} \\ \frac{27}{12} = 2\frac{3}{12} = 2\frac{1}{4}$$

The LCD for these fractions is 12. Change $\frac{5}{6}$ to $\frac{10}{12}$, $\frac{2}{3}$ to $\frac{8}{12}$, and $\frac{3}{4}$ to $\frac{9}{12}$. Add the numerators. The answer is $\frac{27}{12}$. Turn this improper fraction into a mixed number and reduce.

Thus, $\frac{5}{6} + \frac{2}{3} + \frac{3}{4} = 2\frac{1}{4}$

EXERCISES IN ADDING FRACTIONS WITH UNLIKE DENOMINATORS

(Answers are on page 44.)

1) $\dfrac{1}{6}$
   $+\dfrac{2}{3}$

2) $\dfrac{1}{4}$
   $+\dfrac{3}{8}$

3) $\dfrac{1}{2}$
   $+\dfrac{3}{4}$

4) $\dfrac{6}{15}$
   $+\dfrac{3}{5}$

5) $\dfrac{1}{3}$
   $+\dfrac{3}{8}$

6) $\dfrac{3}{5}$
   $+\dfrac{1}{3}$

7) $\dfrac{1}{6}$
$+\dfrac{1}{4}$

8) $\dfrac{2}{3}$
$+\dfrac{4}{7}$

9) $\dfrac{5}{6}$
$+\dfrac{3}{4}$

10) $\dfrac{1}{2}$
$\dfrac{1}{4}$
$+\dfrac{1}{6}$

11) $\dfrac{5}{6}$
$\dfrac{2}{3}$
$+\dfrac{1}{2}$

12) $\dfrac{2}{3}$
$\dfrac{2}{3}$
$+\dfrac{5}{6}$

ADDING MIXED NUMBERS WITH LIKE DENOMINATORS

To add mixed numbers with like denominators, add the fractions and the whole numbers separately. If the fraction part of the answer is an improper fraction, change it to a mixed number and add the whole numbers. Reduce if possible.

Example 7

7a) *Add* $3\frac{1}{7} + 2\frac{3}{7}$

$$3\frac{1}{7}$$
$$+2\frac{3}{7}$$
$$\overline{5\frac{4}{7}}$$

Add the numerators: $1 + 3 = 4$. The answer is $\frac{4}{7}$
Add the whole numbers: $3 + 2 = 5$. The fraction part of the answer is a proper fraction and need not be reduced.

Thus, $3\frac{1}{7} + 2\frac{3}{7} = 5\frac{4}{7}$

7b) *Add* $2\frac{7}{12} + 4\frac{5}{12}$

$$2\frac{7}{12}$$
$$+4\frac{5}{12}$$
$$\overline{6\frac{12}{12}} = 6 + 1 = 7$$

Add the numerators: $7 + 5 = 12$. The answer is $\frac{12}{12}$.
Add the whole numbers: $2 + 4 = 6$. The fraction part of the answer is equal to 1. Add $1 + 6 = 7$.

Thus, $2\frac{7}{12} + 4\frac{5}{12} = 7$

7c) *Add* $5\frac{7}{16} = 2\frac{13}{16}$

$$5\frac{7}{16}$$
$$+2\frac{13}{16}$$
$$\overline{7\frac{20}{16}} = 7 + 1\frac{4}{16} = 8\frac{1}{4}$$

Add the numerators: $7 + 13 = 20$. The answer is $\frac{20}{16}$.
Add the whole numbers: $5 + 2 = 7$. Turn the improper fraction $\frac{20}{16}$ into a mixed number. Add the whole numbers and reduce the fraction to $\frac{1}{4}$.

Thus, $5\frac{7}{16} = 2\frac{13}{16} = 8\frac{1}{4}$

EXERCISES IN ADDING MIXED NUMBERS WITH LIKE DENOMINATORS

(Answers are on page 45.)

Add these mixed numbers. Change any improper fractions in the answers to mixed numbers. Reduce if possible

1) $3\frac{2}{7}$

$+1\frac{3}{7}$

2) $2\frac{3}{10}$

$+1\frac{1}{10}$

3) $7\frac{5}{16}$

$+6\frac{3}{16}$

4) $6\frac{10}{11}$

$+4\frac{9}{11}$

5) $1\frac{7}{10}$

$1\frac{3}{10}$

$+1\frac{1}{10}$

6) $5\frac{4}{5}$

$2\frac{2}{5}$

$+3\frac{4}{5}$

ADDING MIXED NUMBERS WITH UNLIKE DENOMINATORS

> To add mixed numbers with unlike denominators, follow these steps.
>
> Step 1: Change the fractions so they have like denominators.
>
> Step 2: Next, add the fractions and the whole numbers separately. If the fraction part of the answer is an improper fraction, change it to a mixed number and add the whole numbers. Reduce if possible.

Example 8

8a) *Add* $6\frac{1}{2} + 5\frac{2}{3}$

$$6\frac{1}{2} = 6\frac{3}{6}$$
$$+5\frac{2}{3} = 5\frac{4}{6}$$
$$\overline{\qquad\qquad}$$
$$11\frac{7}{6} = 12\frac{1}{6}$$

The LCD for these fractions is 6. Change the fractions to like denominators and add the numerators: 3 + 4 = 7. The answer is $\frac{7}{6}$. Add the whole numbers: 6 + 5 = 11. Turn the improper fraction into a mixed number and add the whole numbers.

Thus, $6\frac{1}{2} + 5\frac{2}{3} = 12\frac{1}{6}$

8b) *Add* $1\frac{1}{4} + 2\frac{3}{5} + 3\frac{2}{5}$

$$1\frac{1}{4} = 1\frac{5}{20}$$
$$2\frac{3}{5} = 2\frac{12}{20}$$
$$+3\frac{2}{5} = 3\frac{8}{20}$$
$$\overline{\qquad\qquad}$$
$$6\frac{25}{20} = 6 + 1\frac{5}{20} = 7\frac{1}{4}$$

The LCD for these fractions is 20. Change the fractions to like denominators and add the numerators to get $\frac{25}{20}$. Add the whole numbers to get 6. Turn the improper fraction into a mixed number. Add the whole numbers together and reduce the fraction.

Thus, $1\frac{1}{4} + 2\frac{3}{5} + 3\frac{2}{5} = 7\frac{1}{4}$

EXERCISES IN ADDING MIXED NUMBERS WITH UNLIKE DENOMINATORS

(Answers are on pages 45–46.)

Add these mixed numbers. Change any improper fractions to mixed numbers. Reduce if possible.

1) $2\frac{1}{2}$
    $+1\frac{1}{4}$

2) $3\frac{5}{6}$
    $+5\frac{2}{3}$

3) $5\frac{7}{10}$
    $+2\frac{2}{5}$

4) $1\frac{3}{4}$
    $+3\frac{1}{3}$

5) $6\frac{3}{8}$
    $+2\frac{1}{4}$

6) $8\frac{5}{9}$
    $+2\frac{2}{3}$

7) $4\frac{1}{2}$

      $5\frac{2}{3}$

    $+7\frac{3}{4}$
     ———

8) $2\frac{3}{4}$

      $1\frac{3}{5}$

    $+2\frac{2}{3}$
     ———

9) $1\frac{4}{5}$

      $7\frac{9}{10}$

    $+3\frac{1}{2}$
     ———

10) $4\frac{5}{6}$

       $\frac{2}{3}$

     $+2\frac{3}{4}$
      ———

11) $4\frac{1}{5}$

       $3\frac{2}{3}$

     $+2\frac{1}{2}$
      ———

12) $1\frac{4}{5}$

       $1\frac{1}{2}$

     $+1\frac{7}{10}$
      ———

SOLVING ADDITION APPLICATIONS

> Use addition to answer questions that ask for the total or how much something is all together. For the addition process, smaller amounts are combined into a larger amount.
>
> The following key words may indicate the need to add: *total, sum, and, plus, all, altogether, entire, added to,* and *with tax.*
>
> If your answer is an improper fraction, convert it to a mixed number. Reduce if possible. Include the label in the answer.

Example 9

9a) *A patient's chart indicates that she slept $8\frac{3}{4}$ hr at night, $\frac{3}{4}$ hr after breakfast, and $1\frac{1}{2}$ hr after lunch. How many hours did she sleep?*

$$8\frac{3}{4} = 8\frac{3}{4}$$
$$\frac{3}{4} = \frac{3}{4}$$
$$+1\frac{1}{2} = 1\frac{2}{4}$$
$$\overline{\qquad 9\frac{8}{4} = 9 + 2 = 11}$$

This is an addition problem. Add the individual amounts of time to get the total amount the patient slept. Convert the fractions to the same denominator. The fraction part of the answer is an improper fraction. Change it to a whole number. Add the whole numbers together.

Thus, the patient slept a total of 11 hr.

9b) *A patient drank $\frac{2}{3}$ cup of juice and $\frac{3}{4}$ cup of milk for breakfast. What was the patient's fluid intake?*

$$\frac{2}{3} = \frac{8}{12}$$
$$+\frac{3}{4} = \frac{9}{12}$$
$$\overline{\qquad \frac{17}{12} = 1\frac{5}{12}}$$

This is an addition problem. Add the amounts of fluid the patient drank to get the total fluid intake for breakfast. Convert the fractions to the same denominator. Change the improper fraction to a mixed number.

Thus, the patient drank $1\frac{5}{12}$ cups.

EXERCISES IN SOLVING ADDITION APPLICATIONS

(*Answers are on pages 46–47.*)

Use addition to solve these problems.

1) Yesterday, you gave your patient $\frac{3}{4}$ tablespoons (tbsp) of medication with breakfast, $\frac{1}{2}$ tbsp at lunch, $\frac{1}{2}$ tbsp at dinner, and $1\frac{1}{4}$ tbsp at bedtime. How much medication did you give?

2) An infant grew $\frac{3}{4}$ in. during her first month of life. She grew $\frac{1}{2}$ in. the second month, $\frac{7}{8}$ in. the third month, and $1\frac{1}{8}$ in. the fourth month. How much has she grown?

3) A patient weighed $170\frac{1}{2}$ lb at her previous visit. At this visit, she weighs $2\frac{3}{4}$ lb more. How much does she weigh?

4) A nurse worked $9\frac{1}{4}$ hr on Monday, $10\frac{1}{2}$ hr on Tuesday, $8\frac{3}{4}$ on Wednesday, $6\frac{3}{4}$ hr on Thursday, and $10\frac{1}{2}$ hr on Friday. How many hours did the nurse work?

5) A patient received $1\frac{1}{3}$ fl oz of medication at breakfast, $1\frac{1}{4}$ fl oz at lunch, $1\frac{1}{2}$ fl oz at dinner and $1\frac{3}{4}$ fl oz at bedtime. How much medication did the patient receive?

SECTION TEST: ADDITION OF FRACTIONS

(Answers are on pages 48–50.)

1) What is the least common multiple of 4 and 6?

2) What is the least common multiple of 2, 3, and 5?

3) What is the least common multiple of 4, 6, and 8?

Raise each fraction to its equivalent higher term by supplying the missing numerator.

4) $\dfrac{2}{3} = \dfrac{}{21}$

5) $\dfrac{1}{4} = \dfrac{}{16}$

6) $\dfrac{2}{5} = \dfrac{}{45}$

Add these fractions. Change fractions to like denominators when necessary. If the answer is an improper fraction, convert it to a mixed number. Reduce if possible.

7) $\dfrac{3}{12}$

$+\dfrac{5}{12}$

8) $\dfrac{5}{9}$

$+\dfrac{4}{9}$

9) $\dfrac{3}{8}$

$+\dfrac{1}{8}$

10) $\dfrac{5}{6}$

$+\dfrac{1}{3}$

11) $\dfrac{1}{4}$

$+\dfrac{4}{5}$

12) $\dfrac{2}{3}$

$+\dfrac{3}{5}$

13) $2\dfrac{1}{5}$

$+6\dfrac{3}{5}$

14) $5\dfrac{6}{7}$

$+3\dfrac{5}{7}$

15) $4\dfrac{5}{8}$

$+1\dfrac{7}{8}$

16) $7\frac{2}{3}$

$+8\frac{1}{2}$

17) $1\frac{3}{4}$

$+3\frac{2}{3}$

18) $9\frac{5}{6}$

$+2\frac{5}{8}$

19) $4\frac{1}{4}$

$3\frac{1}{3}$

$+2\frac{1}{2}$

20) $1\frac{1}{6}$

$1\frac{1}{4}$

$+1\frac{1}{12}$

21) $5\frac{4}{5}$

$4\frac{1}{4}$

$+3\frac{3}{4}$

Solve these application problems.

22) A nurse worked $10\frac{3}{4}$ hr on Monday, $11\frac{1}{2}$ hr on

Tuesday, and $10\frac{3}{4}$ hr on Wednesday.

How many hours did she work for these three days?

23) A patient drank $6\frac{3}{4}$ oz of juice and $7\frac{1}{2}$ oz of

coffee for breakfast. How many oz of liquid did the patient drink?

24) A resident weighed $162\frac{1}{2}$ lbs on the first of the

month. At the end of the month, the resident

had gained $3\frac{3}{4}$ lb. How much did the resident

weigh at the end of the month?

25) A patient received $1\frac{3}{4}$ oz of medication at 1 pm,

$1\frac{1}{4}$ oz at 2 pm, $\frac{3}{4}$ oz at 3 pm, and $\frac{1}{2}$ oz at 4 pm.

How much medication did the patient receive?

ANSWERS TO EXERCISES IN ADDING FRACTIONS WITH LIKE DENOMINATORS

(*Exercises are on pages 20–21.*)

1) $\frac{4}{11} + \frac{5}{11} = \frac{9}{11}$

2) $\frac{7}{25} + \frac{12}{25} = \frac{19}{25}$

3) $\frac{15}{47} + \frac{15}{47} = \frac{30}{47}$

4) $\frac{3}{5} + \frac{2}{5} = \frac{5}{5} = 1$

5) $\frac{4}{13} + \frac{6}{13} = \frac{10}{13}$

6) $\frac{4}{9} + \frac{7}{9} = \frac{11}{9} = 1\frac{2}{9}$

7) $\frac{2}{15} + \frac{4}{15} + \frac{1}{15} = \frac{7}{15}$

8) $\frac{7}{9} + \frac{2}{9} + \frac{5}{9} = \frac{14}{9} = 1\frac{5}{9}$

9) $\frac{5}{8} + \frac{7}{8} + \frac{3}{8} + \frac{1}{8} = \frac{16}{8} = 2$

10) $\frac{9}{10} + \frac{9}{10} = \frac{18}{10} = 1\frac{8}{10} = 1\frac{4}{5}$

11) $\frac{3}{8} + \frac{7}{8} = \frac{10}{8} = 1\frac{2}{8} = 1\frac{1}{4}$

12) $\frac{5}{12} + \frac{11}{12} = \frac{16}{12} = 1\frac{4}{12} = 1\frac{1}{3}$

ANSWERS TO EXERCISES IN FINDING THE LEAST COMMON MULTIPLE OF A SET OF NUMBERS

(*Exercises are on page 24.*)

1) *What is the least common multiple of 4 and 5?*

Start by listing the multiples of the larger number first.
The multiples of 5: 5, 10, 15, <u>20</u>, 25 …
The multiples of 4: 4, 8, 12, 16, <u>20</u>, 24 …
The least common multiple of 4 and 5 is 20.

2) *What is the least common multiple of 6 and 8?*

The multiples of 8: 8, 16, <u>24</u>, 32 …
The multiples of 6: 6, 12, 18, <u>24</u>, 30 …
The least common multiple of 6 and 8 is 24.

3) *What is the least common multiple of 2, 3, and 5?*

The multiples of 5: 5, 10, 15, 20, 25, <u>30</u>, 35 …
The multiples of 3: 3, 6, 9, 12, 15, 18, 21, 24, 27, <u>30</u>, 33 …
The multiples of 2: 2, 4, 6, 8, 10, 12, 14, 16, 18, 20, 22, 24, 26, 28, <u>30</u>, 32 …
The least common multiple of 2, 3, and 5 is 30.

ANSWERS TO EXERCISES IN RAISING A FRACTION TO A HIGHER TERM

(*Exercises are on page 26.*)

1) $\frac{1}{2} = \frac{3}{6}$ 2) $\frac{2}{3} = \frac{10}{15}$ 3) $\frac{3}{4} = \frac{18}{24}$

4) $\frac{2}{5} = \frac{14}{35}$ 5) $\frac{1}{6} = \frac{3}{18}$ 6) $\frac{4}{7} = \frac{12}{21}$

7) $\frac{3}{10} = \frac{21}{70}$ 8) $\frac{7}{12} = \frac{28}{48}$ 9) $\frac{1}{2} = \frac{8}{16}$

ANSWERS TO EXERCISES IN ADDING FRACTIONS WITH UNLIKE DENOMINATORS

(*Exercises are on pages 29–30.*)

1)
$$\frac{1}{6} = \frac{1}{6}$$
$$+\frac{2}{3} = \frac{4}{6}$$
$$\frac{5}{6}$$

2)
$$\frac{1}{4} = \frac{2}{8}$$
$$+\frac{3}{8} = \frac{3}{8}$$
$$\frac{5}{8}$$

3)
$$\frac{1}{2} = \frac{2}{4}$$
$$+\frac{3}{4} = \frac{3}{4}$$
$$\frac{5}{4} = 1\frac{1}{4}$$

4)
$$\frac{6}{15} = \frac{6}{15}$$
$$+\frac{3}{5} = \frac{9}{15}$$
$$\frac{15}{15} = 1$$

5)
$$\frac{1}{3} = \frac{8}{24}$$
$$+\frac{3}{8} = \frac{9}{24}$$
$$\frac{17}{24}$$

6)
$$\frac{3}{5} = \frac{9}{15}$$
$$+\frac{1}{3} = \frac{5}{15}$$
$$\frac{14}{15}$$

7)
$$\frac{1}{6} = \frac{2}{12}$$
$$+\frac{1}{4} = \frac{3}{12}$$
$$\frac{5}{12}$$

8)
$$\frac{2}{3} = \frac{14}{21}$$
$$+\frac{4}{7} = \frac{12}{21}$$
$$\frac{26}{21} = 1\frac{5}{21}$$

9)
$$\frac{5}{6} = \frac{10}{12}$$
$$+\frac{3}{4} = \frac{9}{12}$$
$$\frac{19}{12} = 1\frac{7}{12}$$

10)
$$\frac{1}{2} = \frac{6}{12}$$
$$\frac{1}{4} = \frac{3}{12}$$
$$+\frac{1}{6} = \frac{2}{12}$$
$$\frac{11}{12}$$

11)
$$\frac{5}{6} = \frac{5}{6}$$
$$\frac{2}{3} = \frac{4}{6}$$
$$+\frac{1}{2} = \frac{3}{6}$$
$$\frac{12}{6} = 2$$

12)
$$\frac{2}{3} = \frac{4}{6}$$
$$\frac{2}{3} = \frac{4}{6}$$
$$+\frac{5}{6} = \frac{5}{6}$$
$$\frac{13}{6} = 2\frac{1}{6}$$

ANSWERS TO EXERCISES IN ADDING MIXED NUMBERS WITH LIKE DENOMINATORS

(Exercises are on page 32.)

1) $3\frac{2}{7}$
   $+1\frac{3}{7}$
   $\overline{4\frac{5}{7}}$

2) $2\frac{3}{10}$
   $+1\frac{1}{10}$
   $\overline{3\frac{4}{10} = 3\frac{2}{5}}$

3) $7\frac{5}{16}$
   $+6\frac{3}{16}$
   $\overline{13\frac{8}{16} = 13\frac{1}{2}}$

4) $6\frac{10}{11}$
   $+4\frac{9}{11}$
   $\overline{10\frac{19}{11} = 11\frac{8}{11}}$

5) $1\frac{7}{10}$
   $1\frac{3}{10}$
   $+1\frac{1}{10}$
   $\overline{3\frac{11}{10} = 4\frac{1}{10}}$

6) $5\frac{4}{5}$
   $2\frac{2}{5}$
   $+3\frac{4}{5}$
   $\overline{10\frac{10}{5} = 12}$

ANSWERS TO EXERCISES IN ADDING MIXED NUMBERS WITH UNLIKE DENOMINATORS

(Exercises are on pages 34–35.)

1) $2\frac{1}{2} = 2\frac{2}{4}$
   $+1\frac{1}{4} = 1\frac{1}{4}$
   $\overline{3\frac{3}{4}}$

2) $3\frac{5}{6} = 3\frac{5}{6}$
   $+5\frac{2}{3} = 5\frac{4}{6}$
   $\overline{8\frac{9}{6} = 9\frac{3}{6} = 9\frac{1}{2}}$

3) $5\frac{7}{10} = 5\frac{7}{10}$
   $+2\frac{2}{5} = 2\frac{4}{10}$
   $\overline{7\frac{11}{10} = 8\frac{1}{10}}$

4) $1\frac{3}{4} = 1\frac{9}{12}$
   $+3\frac{1}{3} = 3\frac{4}{12}$
   $\overline{4\frac{13}{12} = 5\frac{1}{12}}$

5) $6\frac{3}{8} = 6\frac{3}{8}$
   $+2\frac{1}{4} = 2\frac{2}{8}$
   $\overline{8\frac{5}{8}}$

6) $8\frac{5}{9} = 8\frac{5}{9}$
   $+2\frac{2}{3} = 2\frac{6}{9}$
   $\overline{10\frac{11}{9} = 11\frac{2}{9}}$

7) $4\frac{1}{2} = 4\frac{6}{12}$

$5\frac{2}{3} = 5\frac{8}{12}$

$+7\frac{3}{4} = 7\frac{9}{12}$

$16\frac{23}{12} = 17\frac{11}{12}$

8) $2\frac{3}{4} = 2\frac{45}{60}$

$1\frac{3}{5} = 1\frac{36}{60}$

$+2\frac{2}{3} = 2\frac{40}{60}$

$5\frac{121}{60} = 7\frac{1}{60}$

9) $1\frac{4}{5} = 1\frac{8}{10}$

$7\frac{9}{10} = 7\frac{9}{10}$

$+3\frac{1}{2} = 3\frac{5}{10}$

$11\frac{22}{10} = 13\frac{2}{10} = 13\frac{1}{5}$

10) $4\frac{5}{6} = 4\frac{10}{12}$

$\frac{2}{3} = \frac{8}{12}$

$+2\frac{3}{4} = 2\frac{9}{12}$

$6\frac{27}{12} = 8\frac{3}{12} = 8\frac{1}{4}$

11) $4\frac{1}{5} = 4\frac{6}{30}$

$3\frac{2}{3} = 3\frac{20}{30}$

$+2\frac{1}{2} = 2\frac{15}{30}$

$9\frac{41}{30} = 10\frac{11}{30}$

12) $1\frac{4}{5} = 1\frac{8}{10}$

$1\frac{1}{2} = 1\frac{5}{10}$

$+1\frac{7}{10} = 1\frac{7}{10}$

$3\frac{20}{10} = 5$

ANSWERS TO EXERCISES IN SOLVING ADDITION APPLICATIONS

(*Exercises are on pages 37–38.*)

1) $\frac{3}{4} = \frac{3}{4}$

$\frac{1}{2} = \frac{2}{4}$

$\frac{1}{2} = \frac{2}{4}$

$+1\frac{1}{4} = 1\frac{1}{4}$

$1\frac{8}{4} = 1 + 2 = 3$

Add the tablespoons of medication to get the total amount given to the patient. Convert the improper fraction in the answer to a mixed number and reduce.

The patient was given 3 tbsp of medication.

2)
$$\frac{3}{4} = \frac{6}{8}$$
$$\frac{1}{2} = \frac{4}{8}$$
$$\frac{7}{8} = \frac{7}{8}$$
$$+1\frac{1}{8} = 1\frac{1}{8}$$
$$1\frac{18}{8} = 3\frac{2}{8} = 3\frac{1}{4}$$

Add the fractions of inches the infant grew to get her total growth in this time period. Convert the improper fraction in the answer to a mixed number and reduce.

The infant grew $3\frac{1}{4}$ in.

3)
$$170\frac{1}{2} = 170\frac{2}{4}$$
$$+2\frac{3}{4} = 2\frac{3}{4}$$
$$172\frac{5}{4} = 173\frac{1}{4}$$

Add the patient's previous weight and her additional weight to get how much she weighs now. Convert the improper fraction in the answer to a mixed number.

The patient now weighs $173\frac{1}{4}$ lb.

4)
$$9\frac{1}{4} = 9\frac{1}{4}$$
$$10\frac{1}{2} = 10\frac{2}{4}$$
$$8\frac{3}{4} = 8\frac{3}{4}$$
$$6\frac{3}{4} = 6\frac{3}{4}$$
$$+10\frac{1}{2} = 10\frac{2}{4}$$
$$43\frac{11}{4} = 45\frac{3}{4}$$

Add the number of hours the nurse worked each day to get the total number of hours she worked. Convert the improper fraction in the answer to a mixed number.

The nurse worked $45\frac{3}{4}$ hr.

5)
$$1\frac{1}{3} = 1\frac{4}{12}$$
$$1\frac{1}{4} = 1\frac{3}{12}$$
$$1\frac{1}{2} = 1\frac{6}{12}$$
$$+1\frac{3}{4} = 1\frac{9}{12}$$
$$4\frac{22}{12} = 5\frac{10}{12} = 5\frac{5}{6}$$

Add the fl oz the patient received to get the total medication the patient received. Convert the improper fraction in the answer to a mixed number and reduce.

The patient received a total of $5\frac{5}{6}$ fl oz.

ANSWERS TO SECTION TEST: ADDITION OF FRACTIONS

(Section Test is on pages 39–42.)

1) The least common multiple of 4 and 6 is 12.

   The multiples of 6: 6, <u>12</u>, 18 ...
   The multiples of 4: 4, 8, <u>12</u>, 16 ...

2) The least common multiple of 2, 3, and 5 is 30.

   The multiples of 5: 5, 10, 15, 20, 25, <u>30</u>, 35 ...
   The multiples of 3: 3, 6, 9, 12, 15, 18, 21, 24, 27, <u>30</u>, 33 ...
   The multiples of 2: 2, 4, 6, 8, 10, 12, 14, 16, 18, 20, 22, 24, 26, 28, <u>30</u>, 32 ...

3) The least common multiple of 4, 6, and 8 is 24.

   The multiples of 8: 8, 16, <u>24</u>, 32 ...
   The multiples of 6: 6, 12, 18, <u>24</u>, 30 ...
   The multiples of 4: 4, 8, 12, 16, 20, <u>24</u>, 28 ...

4) $\dfrac{2}{3} = \dfrac{14}{21}$

5) $\dfrac{1}{4} = \dfrac{4}{16}$

6) $\dfrac{2}{5} = \dfrac{18}{45}$

7) $\dfrac{3}{12}$
    $+\dfrac{5}{12}$
    $\dfrac{8}{12} = \dfrac{2}{3}$

8) $\dfrac{5}{9}$
    $+\dfrac{4}{9}$
    $\dfrac{9}{9} = 1$

9) $\dfrac{3}{8}$
    $+\dfrac{1}{8}$
    $\dfrac{4}{8} = \dfrac{1}{2}$

10) $\dfrac{5}{6} = \dfrac{5}{6}$
     $+\dfrac{1}{3} = \dfrac{2}{6}$
     $\dfrac{7}{6} = 1\dfrac{1}{6}$

11) $\dfrac{1}{4} = \dfrac{5}{20}$
     $+\dfrac{4}{5} = \dfrac{16}{20}$
     $\dfrac{21}{20} = 1\dfrac{1}{20}$

12) $\dfrac{2}{3} = \dfrac{10}{15}$
     $+\dfrac{3}{5} = \dfrac{9}{15}$
     $\dfrac{19}{15} = 1\dfrac{4}{15}$

13) $2\frac{1}{5}$

$+6\frac{3}{5}$

$8\frac{4}{5}$

14) $5\frac{6}{7}$

$+3\frac{5}{7}$

$8\frac{11}{7} = 9\frac{4}{7}$

15) $4\frac{5}{8}$

$+1\frac{7}{8}$

$5\frac{12}{8} = 6\frac{4}{8} = 6\frac{1}{2}$

16) $7\frac{2}{3} = 7\frac{4}{6}$

$+8\frac{1}{2} = 8\frac{3}{6}$

$15\frac{7}{6} = 16\frac{1}{6}$

17) $1\frac{3}{4} = 1\frac{9}{12}$

$+3\frac{2}{3} = 3\frac{8}{12}$

$4\frac{17}{12} = 5\frac{5}{12}$

18) $9\frac{5}{6} = 9\frac{20}{24}$

$+2\frac{5}{8} = 2\frac{15}{24}$

$11\frac{35}{24} = 12\frac{11}{24}$

19) $4\frac{1}{4} = 4\frac{3}{12}$

$3\frac{1}{3} = 3\frac{4}{12}$

$+2\frac{1}{2} = 2\frac{6}{12}$

$9\frac{13}{12} = 10\frac{1}{12}$

20) $1\frac{1}{6} = 1\frac{2}{12}$

$1\frac{1}{4} = 1\frac{3}{12}$

$+1\frac{1}{12} = 1\frac{1}{12}$

$3\frac{6}{12} = 3\frac{1}{2}$

21) $5\frac{4}{5} = 5\frac{16}{20}$

$4\frac{1}{4} = 4\frac{5}{20}$

$+3\frac{3}{4} = 3\frac{15}{20}$

$12\frac{36}{20} = 13\frac{4}{5}$

22) $10\frac{3}{4} = 10\frac{3}{4}$

$11\frac{1}{2} = 11\frac{2}{4}$

$+10\frac{3}{4} = 10\frac{3}{4}$

$31\frac{8}{4} = 33$

Add the number of hours the nurse worked each day to get her total number of hours. Change the fractions to fourths. Convert the improper fraction in the answer to a mixed number. The nurse worked 33 hours.

23) $6\frac{3}{4} = 6\frac{3}{4}$

$+7\frac{1}{2} = 7\frac{2}{4}$

$13\frac{5}{4} = 14\frac{1}{4}$

Add the oz of juice and coffee to get how many oz of liquids the patient drank. Convert the improper fraction in the answer to a mixed number. The patient drank $14\frac{1}{4}$ oz.

24) $162\frac{1}{2} = 162\frac{2}{4}$

$\underline{+3\frac{3}{4} = \quad 3\frac{3}{4}}$

$\qquad 165\frac{5}{4} = 166\frac{1}{4}$

Add the resident's weight at the first of the month and the amount the resident gained to get the resident's total weight at the end of the month.

The resident weighed $166\frac{1}{4}$ lb.

25) $1\frac{3}{4} = 1\frac{3}{4}$

$1\frac{1}{4} = 1\frac{1}{4}$

$\frac{3}{4} = \frac{3}{4}$

$\underline{+\frac{1}{2} = \quad \frac{2}{4}}$

$\qquad 2\frac{9}{4} = 4\frac{1}{4}$

Add the oz of medication the patient received to get the total amount of medication given.

The patient received $4\frac{1}{4}$ oz of medication.

Subtraction of Fractions

OBJECTIVES

Upon completion of this section, you should be able to:

1) Subtract fractions with like denominators.

2) Check a subtraction problem using addition.

3) Subtract fractions with unlike denominators.

4) Subtract a fraction from a whole number using borrowing.

5) Subtract mixed numbers using borrowing.

6) Solve application problems using subtraction.

SUBTRACTING FRACTIONS WITH LIKE DENOMINATORS

The answer to a subtraction problem is called the **difference**. To subtract fractions with the same denominators, subtract the numerators and put the difference in the numerator over the same denominator. Check the answer by using addition.

Example 1

Subtract $\frac{1}{7}$ from $\frac{6}{7}$

$$\begin{array}{r} \frac{6}{7} \\ -\frac{1}{7} \\ \hline \frac{5}{7} \end{array}$$

To subtract $\frac{1}{7}$ from $\frac{6}{7}$, subtract the numerator 1 from 6 to get a difference of 5. Use 5 as the numerator over the original denominator of 7.

Thus, $\frac{6}{7} - \frac{1}{7} = \frac{5}{7}$

To check the answer, add the difference $\left(\frac{5}{7}\right)$ and the number that was subtracted $\left(\frac{1}{7}\right)$ to get the original number: $\frac{5}{7} + \frac{1}{7} = \frac{6}{7}$

Example 2

Subtract $\frac{1}{8}$ from $\frac{7}{8}$

$$\begin{array}{r} \frac{7}{8} \\ -\frac{1}{8} \\ \hline \frac{6}{8} = \frac{3}{4} \end{array}$$

Subtract the numerators $(7 - 1)$ and put the difference (6) over the original denominator (8). Reduce the answer.

Thus, $\frac{7}{8} - \frac{1}{8} = \frac{3}{4}$

Check the answer using addition: $\frac{6}{8} + \frac{1}{8} = \frac{7}{8}$

EXERCISES IN SUBTRACTING FRACTIONS WITH LIKE DENOMINATORS

(*Answers are on page 76.*)

Subtract these fractions. Reduce if possible. Check your answer with addition.

1) $\dfrac{9}{13}$ $-\dfrac{4}{13}$

2) $\dfrac{17}{21}$ $-\dfrac{10}{21}$

3) $\dfrac{16}{25}$ $-\dfrac{11}{25}$

4) $\dfrac{13}{16}$ $-\dfrac{5}{16}$

5) $\dfrac{9}{10}$ $-\dfrac{3}{10}$

6) $\dfrac{17}{24}$ $-\dfrac{9}{24}$

SUBTRACTING FRACTIONS WITH UNLIKE DENOMINATORS

> To subtract fractions with unlike denominators, follow these steps.
>
> Step 1: Find the lowest common denominator for the fractions.
>
> Step 2: Change one or more of the fractions so the fractions all have the same denominator.
>
> Step 3: Subtract the fractions.

Example 3

3a) *Subtract $\frac{1}{8}$ from $\frac{3}{4}$*

$$\frac{3}{4} = \frac{6}{8}$$
$$-\frac{1}{8} = \frac{1}{8}$$
$$\frac{5}{8}$$

Change both fractions to the same denominator. Subtract the numerators.

Thus, $\frac{3}{4} - \frac{1}{8} = \frac{5}{8}$

Check the answer using addition: $\frac{5}{8} + \frac{1}{8} = \frac{6}{8} = \frac{3}{4}$

3b) *Subtract $\frac{7}{12}$ from $\frac{5}{6}$*

$$\frac{5}{6} = \frac{10}{12}$$
$$-\frac{7}{12} = \frac{7}{12}$$
$$\frac{3}{12} = \frac{1}{4}$$

Change both fractions to the same denominator. Subtract the numerators.

Thus, $\frac{5}{6} - \frac{7}{12} = \frac{1}{4}$

Check the answer using addition: $\frac{3}{12} + \frac{7}{12} = \frac{10}{12} = \frac{5}{6}$

EXERCISES IN SUBTRACTING FRACTIONS WITH UNLIKE DENOMINATORS

(Answers are on pages 76–77.)

Subtract these fractions. Reduce if possible. Check your answer with addition.

1) $\frac{7}{8}$
$-\frac{1}{4}$

2) $\frac{1}{2}$
$-\frac{1}{4}$

3) $\frac{2}{3}$
$-\frac{1}{2}$

4) $\frac{3}{4}$
$-\frac{1}{8}$

5) $\frac{4}{5}$
$-\frac{2}{3}$

6) $\frac{5}{7}$
$-\frac{1}{3}$

7) $\frac{4}{9}$
$-\frac{1}{6}$

8) $\frac{1}{3}$
$-\frac{1}{4}$

9) $\frac{2}{3}$
$-\frac{3}{8}$

10) $\frac{13}{15}$
$-\frac{2}{5}$

11) $\frac{2}{3}$
$-\frac{5}{12}$

12) $\frac{9}{16}$
$-\frac{1}{4}$

SUBTRACTING MIXED NUMBERS WITH UNLIKE DENOMINATORS

> To subtract mixed numbers with unlike denominators, follow these steps.
>
> Step 1: Find the lowest common denominator for the fractions.
>
> Step 2: Change one or more of the fractions so they have the same denominator.
>
> Step 3: Subtract the fractions and subtract the whole numbers.

Example 4

4a) *Subtract $2\frac{1}{4}$ from $5\frac{5}{8}$*

$$5\frac{5}{8} = 5\frac{5}{8}$$
$$-2\frac{1}{4} = 2\frac{2}{8}$$
$$\overline{\phantom{-2\frac{1}{4} = }3\frac{3}{8}}$$

Change both fractions to the same denominator. Subtract the numerators. Then, subtract the whole numbers.

Thus, $5\frac{5}{8} - 2\frac{1}{4} = 3\frac{3}{8}$

Check the answer using addition: $3\frac{3}{8} + 2\frac{2}{8} = 5\frac{5}{8}$

4b) *Subtract $8\frac{1}{3}$ from $14\frac{3}{5}$*

$$14\frac{3}{5} = 14\frac{9}{15}$$
$$-\ 8\frac{1}{3} = \ 8\frac{5}{15}$$
$$\overline{\phantom{-\ 8\frac{1}{3} = }6\frac{4}{15}}$$

Change both fractions to the same denominator. Subtract the numerators. Next, subtract the whole numbers.

Thus, $14\frac{3}{5} - 8\frac{1}{3} = 6\frac{4}{15}$

Check the answer using addition: $6\frac{4}{15} + 8\frac{5}{15} = 14\frac{9}{15} = 14\frac{3}{5}$

EXERCISES IN SUBTRACTING MIXED NUMBERS
WITH UNLIKE DENOMINATORS

(Answers are on page 77.)

Subtract these mixed numbers. Reduce if possible. Check your answer with addition.

1) $\begin{aligned} 9\frac{7}{8} \\ -7\frac{1}{2} \\ \hline \end{aligned}$

2) $\begin{aligned} 6\frac{1}{2} \\ -1\frac{1}{4} \\ \hline \end{aligned}$

3) $\begin{aligned} 7\frac{2}{3} \\ -6\frac{2}{9} \\ \hline \end{aligned}$

4) $\begin{aligned} 19\frac{3}{4} \\ -15\frac{3}{8} \\ \hline \end{aligned}$

5) $\begin{aligned} 21\frac{4}{5} \\ -14\frac{7}{10} \\ \hline \end{aligned}$

6) $\begin{aligned} 13\frac{5}{7} \\ -9\frac{1}{3} \\ \hline \end{aligned}$

7) $\begin{aligned} 7\frac{13}{16} \\ -5\frac{3}{8} \\ \hline \end{aligned}$

8) $\begin{aligned} 20\frac{4}{5} \\ -16\frac{7}{10} \\ \hline \end{aligned}$

9) $\begin{aligned} 39\frac{5}{8} \\ -13\frac{1}{3} \\ \hline \end{aligned}$

10) $\begin{aligned} 9\frac{11}{12} \\ -1\frac{1}{4} \\ \hline \end{aligned}$

11) $\begin{aligned} 8\frac{2}{3} \\ -2\frac{3}{8} \\ \hline \end{aligned}$

12) $\begin{aligned} 3\frac{3}{4} \\ -3\frac{2}{3} \\ \hline \end{aligned}$

CONVERTING 1 TO A FRACTION WITH A SPECIFIC DENOMINATOR

> To convert 1 to a fraction with a specific denominator, follow these steps.
>
> Step 1:   Change 1 to a fraction of $\frac{1}{1}$
>
> Step 2:   Raise this fraction to a fraction with the denominator needed. If the denominator needed is 3, then the fraction becomes $\frac{3}{3}$

Example 5

5a) *Change* 1 *to* $\frac{}{5}$

$1 = \frac{1}{1} = \frac{5}{5}$

5b) *Change* 1 *to* $\frac{}{9}$

$1 = \frac{1}{1} = \frac{9}{9}$

5c) *Change* 1 *to* $\frac{}{8}$

$1 = \frac{1}{1} = \frac{8}{8}$

5d) *Change* 1 *to* $\frac{}{15}$

$1 = \frac{1}{1} = \frac{15}{15}$

EXERCISES IN CONVERTING 1 TO A FRACTION WITH A SPECIFIC DENOMINATOR

(Answers are on page 78.)

Convert 1 to the fraction indicated.

1) $1 = \dfrac{}{3}$

2) $1 = \dfrac{}{12}$

3) $1 = \dfrac{}{16}$

4) $1 = \dfrac{}{24}$

5) $1 = \dfrac{}{35}$

6) $1 = \dfrac{}{50}$

SUBTRACTING A FRACTION FROM A WHOLE NUMBER

> To subtract a fraction from a whole number, follow these steps.
>
> Step 1: Borrow 1 from the whole number and change it to a fraction, creating a mixed number.
>
> Step 2: Change the fraction so it has the same denominator as the fraction to be subtracted.
>
> Step 3: Subtract the fraction from the mixed number.

Example 6

6a) *Subtract $\frac{2}{3}$ from 4*

$$4 = 3 + \frac{1}{1} = 3\frac{3}{3}$$
$$-\ \frac{2}{3} = \qquad = \frac{2}{3}$$
$$\overline{\qquad\qquad 3\frac{1}{3}}$$

Thus, $4 - \frac{2}{3} = 3\frac{1}{3}$

Check the answer using addition: $3\frac{1}{3} + \frac{2}{3} = 4$

6b) *Subtract $\frac{7}{12}$ from 6*

$$6 = 5 + \frac{1}{1} = 5\frac{12}{12}$$
$$-\ \frac{7}{12} = \qquad\qquad \frac{7}{12}$$
$$\overline{\qquad\qquad 5\frac{5}{12}}$$

Thus, $6 - \frac{7}{12} = 5\frac{5}{12}$

Check the answer using addition: $5\frac{5}{12} + \frac{7}{12} = 6$

EXERCISES IN SUBTRACTING A FRACTION FROM A WHOLE NUMBER

(Answers are on page 78.)

Subtract the fraction from the whole number. Check your answer with addition.

1)　　4
　　$-\dfrac{3}{4}$

2)　　9
　　$-\dfrac{3}{5}$

3)　　15
　　$-\dfrac{5}{9}$

4)　　10
　　$-\dfrac{7}{12}$

5)　　3
　　$-\dfrac{10}{21}$

6)　　8
　　$-\dfrac{9}{16}$

BORROWING 1 FROM A MIXED NUMBER

To borrow 1 from a mixed number, follow these steps.

Step 1: Borrow 1 from the whole number.

Step 2: Change the one you borrowed to the same denominator as the fraction in the mixed number.

Step 3: Add the two fractions together.

Example 7

7a) *Borrow* 1 *from* $5\frac{3}{8}$

Step 1: Borrow 1 from 5. The 5 becomes 4 plus the 1 borrowed.

Step 2: Change the 1 borrowed to eighths, because the fraction is eighths. The 1 borrowed becomes $\frac{8}{8}$

Step 3: Add the two fractions. $\frac{8}{8} + \frac{3}{8} = \frac{11}{8}$

Thus: $5\frac{3}{8} = 4 + \frac{1}{1} + \frac{3}{8} = 4 + \frac{8}{8} + \frac{3}{8} = 4\frac{11}{8}$

7b) *Borrow* 1 *from* $20\frac{9}{16}$

Step 1: Borrow 1 from 20. The 20 becomes 19 plus the 1 borrowed.

Step 2: Change the 1 borrowed to sixteenths, because the fraction is sixteenths. The 1 borrowed becomes $\frac{16}{16}$

Step 3: Add the two fractions. $\frac{16}{16} + \frac{9}{16} = \frac{25}{16}$

Thus: $20\frac{9}{16} = 19 + \frac{1}{1} + \frac{9}{16} = 19 + \frac{16}{16} + \frac{9}{16} = 19\frac{25}{16}$

EXERCISES IN BORROWING 1 FROM A MIXED NUMBER

(Answers are on page 78.)

Borrow 1 from each of these mixed numbers.

1) $5\frac{1}{3}$

2) $2\frac{4}{7}$

3) $9\frac{1}{8}$

4) $4\frac{5}{16}$

5) $8\frac{3}{4}$

6) $1\frac{1}{2}$

SUBTRACTING FRACTIONS USING BORROWING

> To subtract fractions using borrowing, follow these steps.
>
> Step 4: Change both fractions to the same denominator if necessary.
>
> Step 5: Borrow 1 from the whole number and change it to the same denominator as the fraction in the mixed number. Add the two fractions together.
>
> Step 6: Subtract the fractions and the whole numbers.

Example 8

8a) *Subtract* $2\frac{4}{5}$ *from* $7\frac{1}{5}$

Step 1: Because both fractions have the same denominator, no changes need be made.

Step 2: Because the fractions cannot be subtracted as they are, borrow 1 from 7 and convert it to the same denominator. Add those two fractions.

$$7\frac{1}{5} = 6 + \frac{1}{1} + \frac{1}{5} = 6 + \frac{5}{5} + \frac{1}{5} = 6\frac{6}{5}$$

Step 3: Subtract the mixed numbers.

$$7\frac{1}{5} = 6\frac{6}{5}$$
$$-2\frac{4}{5} = 2\frac{4}{5}$$
$$\overline{\qquad 4\frac{2}{5}}$$

Thus: $7\frac{1}{5} - 2\frac{4}{5} = 4\frac{2}{5}$

Check the answer using addition: $4\frac{2}{5} + 2\frac{4}{5} = 6\frac{6}{5} = 7\frac{1}{5}$

8b) *Subtract* $5\frac{4}{5}$ *from* $6\frac{3}{10}$

Step 1: One fraction must be changed so that both fractions have the same denominator. $5\frac{4}{5} = 5\frac{8}{10}$

Step 2: The fractions cannot be subtracted as they are, so borrow 1 from 6.

$$6\frac{3}{10} = 5 + \frac{1}{1} + \frac{3}{10} = 5 + \frac{10}{10} + \frac{3}{10} = 5\frac{13}{10}$$

Step 3: Subtract the mixed numbers and reduce the answer.

$$6\frac{3}{10} = 5\frac{13}{10}$$
$$-5\frac{8}{10} = 5\frac{8}{10}$$
$$\overline{\phantom{-5\frac{8}{10} = }\;\frac{5}{10} = \frac{1}{2}}$$

Thus: $6\frac{3}{10} - 5\frac{4}{5} = \frac{1}{2}$

Check the answer using addition: $\frac{5}{10} + 5\frac{8}{10} = 5\frac{13}{10} = 6\frac{3}{10}$

8c) *Subtract* $5\frac{3}{4}$ *from* $9\frac{2}{3}$

Step 1: Change both fractions to the same denominator of 12:

$$9\frac{2}{3} = 9\frac{8}{12} \text{ and } 5\frac{3}{4} = 5\frac{9}{12}$$

Step 2: The fractions cannot be subtracted as is, so borrow 1 from 9.

$$9\frac{8}{12} = 8 + \frac{1}{1} + \frac{8}{12} = 8 + \frac{12}{12} + \frac{8}{12} = 8\frac{20}{12}$$

Step 3: Subtract the mixed numbers.

$$9\frac{2}{3} = 9\frac{8}{12} = 8\frac{20}{12}$$
$$-5\frac{3}{4} = 5\frac{9}{12} = 5\frac{9}{12}$$
$$\overline{\phantom{-5\frac{3}{4} = 5\frac{9}{12} = }\;3\frac{11}{12}}$$

Thus: $9\frac{2}{3} - 5\frac{3}{4} = 3\frac{11}{12}$

Check the answer using addition: $3\frac{11}{12} + 5\frac{9}{12} = 8\frac{20}{12} = 9\frac{8}{12} = 9\frac{2}{3}$

EXERCISES IN SUBTRACTING FRACTIONS USING BORROWING

(Answers are on pages 78–79.)

Subtract these mixed numbers. Check your answer with addition.

1) $\quad 8\frac{1}{3}$

$\quad -1\frac{2}{3}$

2) $\quad 9\frac{1}{5}$

$\quad -6\frac{3}{5}$

3) $\quad 5\frac{1}{12}$

$\quad -3\frac{5}{12}$

4) $\quad 6\frac{2}{9}$

$\quad -2\frac{4}{9}$

5) $\quad 3\frac{3}{10}$

$\quad -1\frac{7}{10}$

6) $\quad 9\frac{1}{4}$

$\quad -\frac{3}{4}$

7) $\begin{array}{r} 5\frac{1}{2} \\ -3\frac{3}{4} \\ \hline \end{array}$

8) $\begin{array}{r} 6\frac{1}{4} \\ -2\frac{5}{8} \\ \hline \end{array}$

9) $\begin{array}{r} 3\frac{1}{6} \\ -1\frac{2}{3} \\ \hline \end{array}$

10) $\begin{array}{r} 5\frac{1}{3} \\ -1\frac{7}{12} \\ \hline \end{array}$

11) $\begin{array}{r} 3\frac{1}{2} \\ -2\frac{3}{5} \\ \hline \end{array}$

12) $\begin{array}{r} 1 \\ -\frac{4}{7} \\ \hline \end{array}$

13) $\begin{array}{r} 7\frac{1}{3} \\ -3\frac{3}{4} \\ \hline \end{array}$

14) $\begin{array}{r} 7\frac{1}{5} \\ -1\frac{3}{4} \\ \hline \end{array}$

15) $\begin{array}{r} 2\frac{1}{6} \\ -1\frac{1}{4} \\ \hline \end{array}$

SOLVING SUBTRACTION APPLICATIONS

> Use subtraction to answer questions that ask for the difference between two numbers. For the subtraction process, a smaller amount is removed from the original amount.
>
> The following key words may indicate the need to subtract: *how much greater than*; *how much less than*; *how much of an increase or decrease*; *how many more*; *how much farther*, or *bigger*, or *smaller*, or *heavier*, and so on.
>
> If your answer is an improper fraction, convert it to a mixed number. Reduce if possible. Include the label in the answer.

Example 9

A nurse has worked $2\frac{3}{4}$ hours of her 8-hour shift. How many hours are left on her shift?

$$
\begin{array}{r}
8 = 7\frac{1}{1} = 7\frac{4}{4} \\
-2\frac{3}{4} = \quad 2\frac{3}{4} \\
\hline
5\frac{1}{4}
\end{array}
$$

Subtract the hours the nurse has already worked $\left(2\frac{3}{4}\right)$ from the total hours of her shift (8). Borrow 1 from 8 and convert it to a fraction with a denominator of 4. Then, do the subtraction.

Thus, the nurse has $5\frac{1}{4}$ hours left to work on her shift.

Check the answer using addition: $5\frac{1}{4} + 2\frac{3}{4} = 7\frac{4}{4} = 8$

Example 10

A patient drank $4\frac{3}{4}$ oz of prune juice from a glass containing $6\frac{1}{2}$ oz. How much prune juice was left?

$$
\begin{array}{r}
6\frac{1}{2} = 6\frac{2}{4} = 5\frac{6}{4} \\
-4\frac{3}{4} = \quad 4\frac{3}{4} \\
\hline
1\frac{3}{4}
\end{array}
$$

This is a subtraction problem. Subtract what the patient drank $(4\frac{3}{4}$ oz) from the total amount in the glass ($6\frac{1}{2}$ oz). Make the denominators the same, and then borrow 1 from $6\frac{1}{2}$ and change it into a fraction with a denominator of 4. Then, do the subtraction.

Thus, there are $1\frac{3}{4}$ oz of juice left in the glass.

Check the answer using addition: $1\frac{3}{4} + 4\frac{3}{4} = 5\frac{6}{4} = 5 + 1\frac{2}{4} = 6\frac{2}{4} = 6\frac{1}{2}$

EXERCISES IN SOLVING SUBTRACTION APPLICATIONS

(*Answers are on page 80.*)

1) A doctor prescribed $1\frac{1}{2}$ oz of powdered medication dissolved in water for a patient. The patient was given $\frac{3}{4}$ oz of medication. How much more medication must be given to the patient?

2) If $6\frac{1}{4}$ oz of a 12-oz bottle of orange juice was poured into a glass, how much orange juice remains in the bottle?

3) Last month a baby grew $\frac{5}{8}$ in. This month the baby grew $\frac{3}{4}$ in. How much more did the baby grow this month compared to last month?

4) A $137\frac{1}{2}$ lb resident lost $6\frac{3}{4}$ lbs due to a recent illness. How much does the resident now weigh?

5) If $\frac{5}{8}$ of a shipment of linens delivered to the hospital was stored in the main linen closet, how much is left to be stored?

6) If $9\frac{2}{3}$ oz is removed from a $13\frac{1}{4}$ oz bottle, how much is left?

EXERCISES IN SOLVING MIXED APPLICATIONS

(Answers are on page 81.)

Solve these application problems using addition and/or subtraction.

1) A large container holds $18\frac{1}{2}$ oz of saline solution. If $6\frac{2}{3}$ oz and $5\frac{3}{4}$ oz are removed, how much is left?

2) A doctor prescribed 8 oz of medication for a patient to be administered over 3 hours. If the attendant gave the patient $2\frac{1}{2}$ oz the first hour and $2\frac{1}{3}$ oz the second hour, how much more does the patient need?

3) A resident in a nursing home who weighed $81\frac{1}{2}$ kg lost $3\frac{3}{4}$ kg. How much does the resident weigh now?

4) The doctor prescribed 2 km of walking exercise a day for an elderly patient. If the patient walked $\frac{1}{2}$ km after breakfast and $\frac{3}{4}$ km after dinner, how much more does the patient need to walk?

SECTION TEST: SUBTRACTION OF FRACTIONS

(Answers are on pages 82–83.)

Subtract these problems. Borrow when necessary. Reduce your final answer. Check your answer by using addition.

1) $\dfrac{6}{7}$

   $-\dfrac{4}{7}$

2) $\dfrac{9}{11}$

   $-\dfrac{3}{11}$

3) $5\dfrac{3}{4}$

   $-4\dfrac{1}{4}$

4) $\dfrac{7}{8}$

   $-\dfrac{1}{2}$

5) $\dfrac{3}{4}$

   $-\dfrac{1}{3}$

6) $\dfrac{4}{5}$

   $-\dfrac{3}{10}$

7) $7\dfrac{3}{4}$

   $-2\dfrac{3}{8}$

8) $8\dfrac{5}{6}$

   $-1\dfrac{1}{3}$

9) $6\dfrac{2}{3}$

   $-2\dfrac{3}{8}$

10) $\quad 4$

$\quad - \dfrac{3}{7}$

11) $\quad 13$

$\quad - \dfrac{13}{16}$

12) $\quad 1$

$\quad - \dfrac{17}{32}$

13) $\quad 3\dfrac{1}{4}$

$\quad -1\dfrac{3}{4}$

14) $\quad 7\dfrac{2}{7}$

$\quad -5\dfrac{5}{7}$

15) $\quad 16\dfrac{3}{10}$

$\quad -5\dfrac{9}{10}$

16) $\quad 3\dfrac{3}{16}$

$\quad - \dfrac{5}{8}$

17) $\quad 4\dfrac{7}{10}$

$\quad -2\dfrac{4}{5}$

18) $\quad 9\dfrac{1}{3}$

$\quad -2\dfrac{3}{4}$

19) $7\frac{1}{9}$

    $-4\frac{5}{6}$

20) $6\frac{3}{8}$

    $-5\frac{11}{12}$

21) $1\frac{1}{4}$

    $-\frac{3}{8}$

22) An attendant gave a resident 1 cup of tomato juice. The resident drank $\frac{3}{4}$ cup. How much juice remains?

23) At the beginning of an 8-hour shift, there are $5\frac{1}{4}$ bottles of hand sanitizer available. At the end of the shift, $3\frac{1}{2}$ bottles remain. How much was used?

ANSWERS TO EXERCISES IN SUBTRACTING FRACTIONS WITH LIKE DENOMINATORS

(Exercises are on page 53.)

1)
$$\begin{array}{r} \frac{9}{13} \\ -\frac{4}{13} \\ \hline \frac{5}{13} \end{array}$$

2)
$$\begin{array}{r} \frac{17}{21} \\ -\frac{10}{21} \\ \hline \frac{7}{21} = \frac{1}{3} \end{array}$$

3)
$$\begin{array}{r} \frac{16}{25} \\ -\frac{11}{25} \\ \hline \frac{5}{25} = \frac{1}{5} \end{array}$$

4)
$$\begin{array}{r} \frac{13}{16} \\ -\frac{5}{16} \\ \hline \frac{8}{16} = \frac{1}{2} \end{array}$$

5)
$$\begin{array}{r} \frac{9}{10} \\ -\frac{3}{10} \\ \hline \frac{6}{10} = \frac{3}{5} \end{array}$$

6)
$$\begin{array}{r} \frac{17}{24} \\ -\frac{9}{24} \\ \hline \frac{8}{24} = \frac{1}{3} \end{array}$$

ANSWERS TO EXERCISES IN SUBTRACTING FRACTIONS WITH UNLIKE DENOMINATORS

(Exercises are on page 55.)

1)
$$\begin{array}{r} \frac{7}{8} = \frac{7}{8} \\ -\frac{1}{4} = \frac{2}{8} \\ \hline \frac{5}{8} \end{array}$$

2)
$$\begin{array}{r} \frac{1}{2} = \frac{2}{4} \\ -\frac{1}{4} = \frac{1}{4} \\ \hline \frac{1}{4} \end{array}$$

3)
$$\begin{array}{r} \frac{2}{3} = \frac{4}{6} \\ -\frac{1}{2} = \frac{3}{6} \\ \hline \frac{1}{6} \end{array}$$

4)
$$\begin{array}{r} \frac{3}{4} = \frac{6}{8} \\ -\frac{1}{8} = \frac{1}{8} \\ \hline \frac{5}{8} \end{array}$$

5)
$$\begin{array}{r} \frac{4}{5} = \frac{12}{15} \\ -\frac{2}{3} = \frac{10}{15} \\ \hline \frac{2}{15} \end{array}$$

6)
$$\begin{array}{r} \frac{5}{7} = \frac{15}{21} \\ -\frac{1}{3} = \frac{7}{21} \\ \hline \frac{8}{21} \end{array}$$

7)
$$\begin{array}{r} \frac{4}{9} = \frac{8}{18} \\ -\frac{1}{6} = \frac{3}{18} \\ \hline \frac{5}{18} \end{array}$$

8)
$$\begin{array}{r} \frac{1}{3} = \frac{4}{12} \\ -\frac{1}{4} = \frac{3}{12} \\ \hline \frac{1}{12} \end{array}$$

9)
$$\begin{array}{r} \frac{2}{3} = \frac{16}{24} \\ -\frac{3}{8} = \frac{9}{24} \\ \hline \frac{7}{24} \end{array}$$

10) $\dfrac{13}{15} = \dfrac{13}{15}$

    $-\dfrac{2}{5} = \dfrac{6}{15}$

        $\dfrac{7}{15}$

11) $\dfrac{2}{3} = \dfrac{8}{12}$

    $-\dfrac{5}{12} = \dfrac{5}{12}$

        $\dfrac{3}{12} = \dfrac{1}{4}$

12) $\dfrac{9}{16} = \dfrac{9}{16}$

    $-\dfrac{1}{4} = \dfrac{4}{16}$

        $\dfrac{5}{16}$

ANSWERS TO EXERCISES IN SUBTRACTING MIXED NUMBERS WITH UNLIKE DENOMINATORS

(Exercises are on page 57.)

1) $9\dfrac{7}{8} = 9\dfrac{7}{8}$

   $-7\dfrac{1}{2} = 7\dfrac{4}{8}$

        $2\dfrac{3}{8}$

2) $6\dfrac{1}{2} = 6\dfrac{2}{4}$

   $-1\dfrac{1}{4} = 1\dfrac{1}{4}$

        $5\dfrac{1}{4}$

3) $7\dfrac{2}{3} = 7\dfrac{6}{9}$

   $-6\dfrac{2}{9} = 6\dfrac{2}{6}$

        $1\dfrac{4}{9}$

4) $19\dfrac{3}{4} = 19\dfrac{6}{8}$

   $-15\dfrac{3}{8} = 15\dfrac{3}{8}$

        $4\dfrac{3}{8}$

5) $21\dfrac{4}{5} = 21\dfrac{8}{10}$

   $-14\dfrac{7}{10} = 14\dfrac{7}{10}$

        $7\dfrac{1}{10}$

6) $13\dfrac{5}{7} = 13\dfrac{15}{21}$

   $-9\dfrac{1}{3} = 9\dfrac{7}{21}$

        $4\dfrac{8}{21}$

7) $7\dfrac{13}{16} = 7\dfrac{13}{16}$

   $-5\dfrac{3}{8} = 5\dfrac{6}{16}$

        $2\dfrac{7}{16}$

8) $20\dfrac{4}{5} = 20\dfrac{8}{10}$

   $-16\dfrac{7}{10} = 16\dfrac{7}{10}$

        $4\dfrac{1}{10}$

9) $39\dfrac{5}{8} = 39\dfrac{15}{24}$

   $13\dfrac{1}{3} = 13\dfrac{8}{24}$

        $26\dfrac{7}{24}$

10) $9\dfrac{11}{12} = 9\dfrac{11}{12}$

   $-1\dfrac{1}{4} = 1\dfrac{3}{12}$

        $8\dfrac{8}{12} = 8\dfrac{2}{3}$

11) $8\dfrac{2}{3} = 8\dfrac{16}{24}$

   $-2\dfrac{3}{8} = 2\dfrac{9}{24}$

        $6\dfrac{7}{24}$

12) $3\dfrac{3}{4} = 3\dfrac{9}{12}$

   $-3\dfrac{2}{3} = 3\dfrac{8}{12}$

        $\dfrac{1}{12}$

ANSWERS TO EXERCISES IN CONVERTING 1 TO A FRACTION WITH A SPECIFIC DENOMINATOR

(Answers are on page 59.)

1) $1 = \frac{3}{3}$

2) $1 = \frac{12}{12}$

3) $1 = \frac{16}{16}$

4) $1 = \frac{24}{24}$

5) $1 = \frac{35}{35}$

6) $1 = \frac{50}{50}$

ANSWERS TO EXERCISES IN SUBTRACTING A FRACTION FROM A WHOLE NUMBER

(Exercises are on page 61.)

1)
$$
\begin{aligned}
4 &= 3\frac{4}{4} \\
-\frac{3}{4} &= \frac{3}{4} \\
\hline
&\quad 3\frac{1}{4}
\end{aligned}
$$

2)
$$
\begin{aligned}
9 &= 8\frac{5}{5} \\
-\frac{3}{5} &= \frac{3}{5} \\
\hline
&\quad 8\frac{2}{5}
\end{aligned}
$$

3)
$$
\begin{aligned}
15 &= 14\frac{9}{9} \\
-\frac{5}{9} &= \frac{5}{9} \\
\hline
&\quad 14\frac{4}{9}
\end{aligned}
$$

4)
$$
\begin{aligned}
10 &= 9\frac{12}{12} \\
-\frac{7}{12} &= \frac{7}{12} \\
\hline
&\quad 9\frac{5}{12}
\end{aligned}
$$

5)
$$
\begin{aligned}
3 &= 2\frac{21}{21} \\
-\frac{10}{21} &= \frac{10}{21} \\
\hline
&\quad 2\frac{11}{21}
\end{aligned}
$$

6)
$$
\begin{aligned}
8 &= 7\frac{16}{16} \\
-\frac{9}{16} &= \frac{9}{16} \\
\hline
&\quad 7\frac{7}{16}
\end{aligned}
$$

ANSWERS TO EXERCISES IN BORROWING 1 FROM A MIXED NUMBER

(Exercises are on page 63.)

1) $5\frac{1}{3} = 4\frac{4}{3}$

2) $2\frac{4}{7} = 1\frac{11}{7}$

3) $9\frac{1}{8} = 8\frac{9}{8}$

4) $4\frac{5}{16} = 3\frac{21}{16}$

5) $8\frac{3}{4} = 7\frac{7}{4}$

6) $1\frac{1}{2} = \frac{3}{2}$

ANSWERS TO EXERCISES IN SUBTRACTING FRACTIONS USING BORROWING

(Exercises are on pages 66–67.)

1)
$$
\begin{aligned}
8\frac{1}{3} &= 7\frac{4}{3} \\
-1\frac{2}{3} &= 1\frac{2}{3} \\
\hline
&\quad 6\frac{2}{3}
\end{aligned}
$$

2)
$$
\begin{aligned}
9\frac{1}{5} &= 8\frac{6}{5} \\
-6\frac{3}{5} &= 6\frac{3}{5} \\
\hline
&\quad 2\frac{3}{5}
\end{aligned}
$$

3)
$$
\begin{aligned}
5\frac{1}{12} &= 4\frac{13}{12} \\
-3\frac{5}{12} &= 3\frac{5}{12} \\
\hline
&\quad 1\frac{8}{12} = 1\frac{2}{3}
\end{aligned}
$$

4) $6\frac{2}{9} = 5\frac{11}{9}$

$-2\frac{4}{9} = 2\frac{4}{9}$

$\phantom{-2\frac{4}{9} = } 3\frac{7}{9}$

5) $3\frac{3}{10} = 2\frac{13}{10}$

$-1\frac{7}{10} = 1\frac{7}{10}$

$\phantom{-1\frac{7}{10} = } 1\frac{6}{10} = 1\frac{3}{5}$

6) $9\frac{1}{4} = 8\frac{5}{4}$

$-\frac{3}{4} = \frac{3}{4}$

$\phantom{-9\frac{3}{4} = } 8\frac{2}{4} = 8\frac{1}{2}$

7) $5\frac{1}{2} = 5\frac{2}{4} = 4\frac{6}{4}$

$-3\frac{3}{4} = \phantom{5\frac{2}{4} = } 3\frac{3}{4}$

$\phantom{-3\frac{3}{4} = 5\frac{2}{4} = } 1\frac{3}{4}$

8) $6\frac{1}{4} = 6\frac{2}{8} = 5\frac{10}{8}$

$-2\frac{5}{8} = \phantom{6\frac{2}{8} = } 2\frac{5}{8}$

$\phantom{-2\frac{5}{8} = 6\frac{2}{8} = } 3\frac{5}{8}$

9) $3\frac{1}{6} = 3\frac{1}{6} = 2\frac{7}{6}$

$-1\frac{2}{3} = \phantom{3\frac{1}{6} = } 1\frac{4}{6}$

$\phantom{-1\frac{2}{3} = 3\frac{1}{6} = } 1\frac{3}{6} = 1\frac{1}{2}$

10) $5\frac{1}{3} = 5\frac{4}{12} = 4\frac{16}{12}$

$-1\frac{7}{12} = \phantom{5\frac{4}{12} = } 1\frac{7}{12}$

$\phantom{-1\frac{7}{12} = 5\frac{4}{12} = } 3\frac{9}{12} = 3\frac{3}{4}$

11) $3\frac{1}{2} = 3\frac{5}{10} = 2\frac{15}{10}$

$-2\frac{3}{5} = \phantom{3\frac{5}{10} = } 2\frac{6}{10}$

$\phantom{-2\frac{3}{5} = 3\frac{5}{10} = } \frac{9}{10}$

12) $1\phantom{\frac{1}{1}} = \frac{7}{7}$

$-\frac{4}{7} = \frac{4}{7}$

$\phantom{-1\frac{4}{7} = } \frac{3}{7}$

13) $7\frac{1}{3} = 7\frac{4}{12} = 6\frac{16}{12}$

$-3\frac{3}{4} = \phantom{7\frac{4}{12} = } 3\frac{9}{12}$

$\phantom{-3\frac{3}{4} = 7\frac{4}{12} = } 3\frac{7}{12}$

14) $7\frac{1}{5} = 7\frac{4}{20} - 6\frac{24}{20}$

$-1\frac{3}{4} = \phantom{7\frac{4}{20} - } 1\frac{15}{20}$

$\phantom{-1\frac{3}{4} = 7\frac{4}{20} - } 5\frac{9}{20}$

15) $2\frac{1}{6} = 2\frac{2}{12} = 1\frac{14}{12}$

$-1\frac{1}{4} = 1\frac{3}{12} = 1\frac{3}{12}$

$\phantom{-1\frac{1}{4} = 1\frac{3}{12} = } \frac{11}{12}$

ANSWERS TO EXERCISES IN SOLVING SUBTRACTION APPLICATIONS

(Exercises are on pages 69–70.)

1) $1\frac{1}{2} = 1\frac{2}{4} = \frac{6}{4}$

  $-\quad\frac{3}{4} = \qquad \frac{3}{4}$

  _____

  $\qquad\qquad\quad \frac{3}{4}$

Subtract the amount of medication the patient was given from the amount of medication the doctor prescribed to get how much more medication the patient needs. The patient needs $\frac{3}{4}$ oz more medication.

2) $12 \quad = 11\frac{4}{4}$

  $-6\frac{1}{4} = \; 6\frac{1}{4}$

  _____

  $\qquad\quad 5\frac{3}{4}$

Subtract the amount of juice poured into the glass from the total amount in the bottle to get the amount that remains in the bottle. $5\frac{3}{4}$ oz of orange juice remains in the bottle.

3) $\frac{3}{4} = \frac{6}{8}$

  $-\frac{5}{8} = \frac{5}{8}$

  _____

  $\quad \frac{1}{8}$

Subtract the amount the baby grew this month from the amount the baby grew last month to find how much more the baby grew.

The baby grew $\frac{1}{8}$ in. more this month than last month.

4) $137\frac{1}{2} = 137\frac{2}{4} = 136\frac{6}{4}$

  $-\quad 6\frac{3}{4} = \qquad\qquad\; 6\frac{3}{4}$

  _____

  $\qquad\qquad\qquad\quad 130\frac{3}{4}$

Subtract the amount of weight the resident lost from the resident's original weight to find how much the resident now weighs. The resident now weighs $130\frac{3}{4}$ lb.

5) $1 \; = \frac{8}{8}$

  $-\frac{5}{8} = \frac{5}{8}$

  _____

  $\quad \frac{3}{8}$

Subtract the fraction of the shipment that was stored in the linen closet from 1 (because there was 1 shipment) to get the fraction of the shipment that remains to be stored. There is $\frac{3}{8}$ of the shipment that remains to be stored.

6) $13\frac{1}{4} = 13\frac{3}{12} = 12\frac{15}{12}$

  $-\; 9\frac{2}{3} = \; 9\frac{8}{12} = \; 9\frac{8}{12}$

  _____

  $\qquad\qquad\qquad\quad 3\frac{7}{12}$

Subtract the amount that was removed from the original amount in the bottle to find out how much is left. There are $3\frac{7}{12}$ oz left in the bottle.

ANSWERS TO EXERCISES IN SOLVING MIXED APPLICATIONS

(Exercises are on pages 71–72.)

1) This is a multistep problem. Add the amounts of saline solution that were removed from the container. Subtract this from the original amount in the container.

$$6\tfrac{2}{3} = 6\tfrac{8}{12} \qquad\qquad 18\tfrac{1}{2} = 18\tfrac{6}{12}$$
$$+5\tfrac{3}{4} = 5\tfrac{9}{12} \qquad\qquad -12\tfrac{5}{12} = 12\tfrac{5}{12}$$
$$\overline{11\tfrac{17}{12} = 12\tfrac{5}{12}} \qquad\qquad \overline{6\tfrac{1}{12}}$$

There are $6\tfrac{1}{12}$ oz of saline solution left in the container.

2) This is a multistep problem. Add the amount of medication the patient has already been given. Subtract this from the amount of medication the doctor prescribed to find how much more medication the patient needs.

$$2\tfrac{1}{2} = 2\tfrac{3}{6} \qquad\qquad 8 = 7\tfrac{6}{6}$$
$$+2\tfrac{1}{3} - 2\tfrac{2}{6} \qquad\qquad -4\tfrac{5}{6} = 4\tfrac{5}{6}$$
$$\overline{4\tfrac{5}{6}} \qquad\qquad \overline{3\tfrac{1}{6}}$$

The patient needs $3\tfrac{1}{6}$ oz more medication.

3)
$$81\tfrac{1}{2} = 81\tfrac{2}{4} = 80\tfrac{6}{4}$$
$$-\ 3\tfrac{3}{4} = \qquad\quad 3\tfrac{3}{4}$$
$$\overline{\phantom{-3\tfrac{3}{4}=}\ 77\tfrac{3}{4}}$$

This is a subtraction problem. Subtract the amount of weight the resident lost from the resident's original weight to find out how much the resident now weighs.

The resident now weighs $77\tfrac{3}{4}$ kg.

4) This is a multistep problem. Add the number (amount) of km the patient has walked. Subtract this from the number (amount) of km the doctor has prescribed to find the number (amount) of km the patient still needs to walk.

$$\tfrac{1}{2} = \tfrac{2}{4} \qquad\qquad\qquad\qquad 2 = 1\tfrac{4}{4}$$
$$+\tfrac{3}{4} = \tfrac{3}{4} \qquad\qquad\qquad\qquad -1\tfrac{1}{4} = 1\tfrac{1}{4}$$
$$\overline{\tfrac{5}{4} = 1\tfrac{1}{4}} \qquad\qquad\qquad\qquad \overline{\phantom{-1\tfrac{1}{4}=1}\tfrac{3}{4}}$$

The elderly patient needs to walk another $\tfrac{3}{4}$ km.

ANSWERS TO SECTION TEST: SUBTRACTION OF FRACTIONS

(Section Test is on pages 73–75.)

1) $\dfrac{6}{7}$

$-\dfrac{4}{7}$

$\dfrac{2}{7}$

2) $\dfrac{9}{11}$

$-\dfrac{3}{11}$

$\dfrac{6}{11}$

3) $5\dfrac{3}{4}$

$-4\dfrac{1}{4}$

$1\dfrac{2}{4} = 1\dfrac{1}{2}$

4) $\dfrac{7}{8} = \dfrac{7}{8}$

$-\dfrac{1}{2} = \dfrac{4}{8}$

$\dfrac{3}{8}$

5) $\dfrac{3}{4} = \dfrac{9}{12}$

$-\dfrac{1}{3} = \dfrac{4}{12}$

$\dfrac{5}{12}$

6) $\dfrac{4}{5} = \dfrac{8}{10}$

$-\dfrac{3}{10} = \dfrac{3}{10}$

$\dfrac{5}{10} = \dfrac{1}{2}$

7) $7\dfrac{3}{4} = 7\dfrac{6}{8}$

$-2\dfrac{3}{8} = 2\dfrac{3}{8}$

$5\dfrac{3}{8}$

8) $8\dfrac{5}{6} = 8\dfrac{5}{6}$

$-1\dfrac{1}{3} = 1\dfrac{2}{6}$

$7\dfrac{3}{6} = 7\dfrac{1}{2}$

9) $6\dfrac{2}{3} = 6\dfrac{16}{24}$

$-2\dfrac{3}{8} = 2\dfrac{9}{24}$

$4\dfrac{7}{24}$

10) $4 = 3\dfrac{7}{7}$

$-\dfrac{3}{7} = \dfrac{3}{7}$

$3\dfrac{4}{7}$

11) $13 = 12\dfrac{16}{16}$

$-\dfrac{13}{16} = \dfrac{13}{16}$

$12\dfrac{3}{16}$

12) $1 = \dfrac{32}{32}$

$-\dfrac{17}{32} = \dfrac{17}{32}$

$\dfrac{15}{32}$

13) $3\dfrac{1}{4} = 2\dfrac{5}{4}$

$-1\dfrac{3}{4} = 1\dfrac{3}{4}$

$1\dfrac{2}{4} = 1\dfrac{1}{2}$

14) $7\dfrac{2}{7} = 6\dfrac{9}{7}$

$-5\dfrac{5}{7} = 5\dfrac{5}{7}$

$1\dfrac{4}{7}$

15) $16\dfrac{3}{10} = 15\dfrac{13}{10}$

$-5\dfrac{9}{10} = 5\dfrac{9}{10}$

$10\dfrac{4}{10} = 10\dfrac{2}{5}$

16) $3\frac{3}{16} = 3\frac{3}{16} = 2\frac{19}{16}$

$-\frac{5}{8} = \frac{10}{16} = \frac{10}{16}$

$\overline{\qquad\quad 2\frac{9}{16}}$

17) $4\frac{7}{10} = 4\frac{7}{10} = 3\frac{17}{10}$

$-2\frac{4}{5} = 2\frac{8}{10} = 2\frac{8}{10}$

$\overline{\qquad\quad 1\frac{9}{10}}$

18) $9\frac{1}{3} = 9\frac{4}{12} = 8\frac{16}{12}$

$-2\frac{3}{4} = 2\frac{9}{12} = 2\frac{9}{12}$

$\overline{\qquad\quad 6\frac{7}{12}}$

19) $7\frac{1}{9} = 7\frac{2}{18} = 6\frac{20}{18}$

$-4\frac{5}{6} = 4\frac{15}{18} = 4\frac{15}{18}$

$\overline{\qquad\quad 2\frac{5}{18}}$

20) $6\frac{3}{8} = 6\frac{9}{24} = 5\frac{33}{24}$

$-5\frac{11}{12} = 5\frac{22}{24} = 5\frac{22}{24}$

$\overline{\qquad\quad \frac{11}{24}}$

21) $1\frac{1}{4} = 1\frac{2}{8} = \frac{10}{8}$

$-\ \ \frac{3}{8} = \ \ \frac{3}{8} = \ \ \frac{3}{8}$

$\overline{\qquad\quad \frac{7}{8}}$

22) $1\ \ = \frac{4}{4}$

$-\ \ \frac{3}{4} = \frac{3}{4}$

$\overline{\qquad \frac{1}{4}}$

Subtract the amount of tomato juice the resident drank from the total amount the resident was given to find out how much juice remains.

There is $\frac{1}{4}$ cup of tomato juice remaining.

23) $5\frac{1}{4} = 5\frac{1}{4} = 4\frac{5}{4}$

$-3\frac{1}{2} = 3\frac{2}{4} = 3\frac{2}{4}$

$\overline{\qquad\quad 1\frac{3}{4}}$

Subtract the amount of hand sanitizer remaining at the end of this shift from the amount of hand sanitizer available at the beginning of the shift to find out how much was used.

There were $1\frac{3}{4}$ bottles used.

Multiplication of Fractions

OBJECTIVES

Upon completion of this section, you should be able to:

1) Multiply two fractions together.

2) Cancel when multiplying fractions.

3) Multiply a fraction times a whole number.

4) Multiply a fraction times a mixed number.

5) Multiply two mixed numbers together.

6) Solve application problems using multiplication.

MULTIPLYING FRACTIONS

> To multiply two fractions together, multiply the numerators together and multiply the denominators together. Reduce the answer if possible.

Example 1

1a) *Represent* $\frac{1}{2} \times \frac{6}{8}$ *as a diagram.*

Figure 4-1 is divided into 8 sections; each section is $\frac{1}{8}$ of the entire box. The shaded area represents $\frac{6}{8}$ of the entire box.

$\frac{1}{8}$	$\frac{1}{8}$	$\frac{1}{8}$	$\frac{1}{8}$
$\frac{1}{8}$	$\frac{1}{8}$	$\frac{1}{8}$	$\frac{1}{8}$

Figure 4-1

85

Figure 4-2 shows a thick black line around $\frac{1}{2}$ of the shaded boxes. The black line surrounds 3 of the $\frac{1}{8}$ boxes. Thus, $\frac{1}{2} \times \frac{6}{8} = \frac{3}{8}$

$\frac{1}{8}$	$\frac{1}{8}$	$\frac{1}{8}$	$\frac{1}{8}$
$\frac{1}{8}$	$\frac{1}{8}$	$\frac{1}{8}$	$\frac{1}{8}$

Figure 4-2

1b) *Solve $\frac{1}{2} \times \frac{6}{8}$ by multiplying the fractions.*

Step 1:   Multiply the numerators together. 1 times 6 = 6.

Step 2:   Multiply the denominators together. 2 times 8 = 16.

Step 3:   Reduce the numerator and the denominator in the answer by 2.

$$\frac{1}{2} \times \frac{6}{8} = \frac{1 \times 6}{2 \times 8} = \frac{6}{16} = \frac{3}{8}$$

Thus: $\frac{1}{2} \times \frac{6}{8} = \frac{3}{8}$

Example 2

Multiply $\frac{1}{4} \times \frac{1}{3}$

Step 1:   Multiply the numerators together. 1 times 1 = 1.

Step 2:   Multiply the denominators together. 4 times 3 = 12.

Step 3:   This fraction cannot be reduced.

$$\frac{1}{4} \times \frac{1}{3} = \frac{1 \times 1}{4 \times 3} = \frac{1}{12}$$

Thus: $\frac{1}{4} \times \frac{1}{3} = \frac{1}{12}$

Example 3

Multiply $\frac{1}{2} \times \frac{3}{5} \times \frac{3}{4}$

Step 1:   Multiply the numerators together. 1 times 3 times 3 = 9.

Step 2:   Multiply the denominators together. 2 times 5 times 4 = 40.

Step 3:   This fraction cannot be reduced.

$$\frac{1}{2} \times \frac{3}{5} \times \frac{3}{4} = \frac{1 \times 3 \times 3}{2 \times 5 \times 4} = \frac{9}{40}$$

Thus: $\frac{1}{2} \times \frac{3}{5} \times \frac{3}{4} = \frac{9}{40}$

EXERCISES IN MULTIPLYING FRACTIONS

(Answers are on page 104.)

Multiply these fractions. Reduce the answer if possible.

1) $\frac{3}{5} \times \frac{1}{4}$

2) $\frac{5}{9} \times \frac{1}{2}$

3) $\frac{3}{5} \times \frac{6}{7}$

4) $\frac{3}{4} \times \frac{3}{5}$

5) $\frac{1}{2} \times \frac{2}{3}$

6) $\frac{5}{8} \times \frac{3}{4}$

7) $\frac{4}{5} \times \frac{1}{8}$

8) $\frac{3}{4} \times \frac{3}{4}$

9) $\frac{7}{8} \times \frac{5}{7}$

10) $\frac{1}{2} \times \frac{1}{4} \times \frac{3}{4}$

11) $\frac{1}{2} \times \frac{3}{4} \times \frac{3}{5}$

12) $\frac{1}{2} \times \frac{3}{5} \times \frac{1}{2}$

CANCELING WHEN MULTIPLYING FRACTIONS

> Canceling is a method of reducing fractions before they are multiplied. When canceling fractions, reduce any one of the numerators with any one of the denominators. Continue reducing other numerators and denominators until no more reducing can be done. Multiply the fractions.

Example 4

4a) *Use the canceling method to multiply $\frac{1}{4} \times \frac{2}{3}$*

Although $\frac{1}{4}$ and $\frac{2}{3}$ cannot be reduced, the 2 in the numerator of $\frac{2}{3}$ can cancel with the 4 in the denominator of $\frac{1}{4}$. 2 will divide into 2 one time, and 2 will divide into 4 two times.

$$\frac{1}{\overset{}{\underset{2}{4}}} \times \frac{\overset{1}{2}}{3} = \frac{1 \times 1}{2 \times 3} = \frac{1}{6}. \text{ Thus, } \frac{1}{4} \times \frac{2}{3} = \frac{1}{6}$$

4b) *Multiply $\frac{1}{4} \times \frac{2}{3}$ <u>without</u> canceling.*

$$\frac{1}{4} \times \frac{2}{3} = \frac{1 \times 2}{4 \times 3} = \frac{2}{12} = \frac{1}{6}$$

Note: In 4a, the canceling reduces the fractions before the multiplication. In 4b the fraction $\frac{2}{12}$ is reduced after the multiplication. Either way, the answers are the same. If the canceling method is used, the answer will generally not have to be reduced.

Example 5

Use the canceling method to multiply $\frac{5}{8} \times \frac{2}{5}$

Step 1:   Cancel the 5's: $\frac{\overset{1}{5}}{8} \times \frac{2}{\underset{1}{5}}$

Step 2:   Cancel the 8 and 2: $\frac{\overset{1}{5}}{\underset{4}{8}} \times \frac{\overset{1}{2}}{\underset{1}{5}}$

Step 3:   Multiply the fraction: $\frac{\overset{1}{5}}{\underset{4}{8}} \times \frac{\overset{1}{2}}{\underset{1}{5}} = \frac{1 \times 1}{4 \times 1} = \frac{1}{4}$

Thus: $\frac{5}{8} \times \frac{2}{5} = \frac{1}{4}$

Example 6

Use the canceling method to multiply $\frac{3}{10} \times \frac{5}{7} \times \frac{14}{21}$

Step 1: Cancel the 5 and 10: $\frac{3}{\overset{}{\underset{2}{\cancel{10}}}} \times \frac{\overset{1}{\cancel{5}}}{7} \times \frac{14}{21}$

Step 2: Cancel the 7 and 14: $\frac{3}{\underset{2}{\cancel{10}}} \times \frac{\overset{1}{\cancel{5}}}{\underset{1}{\cancel{7}}} \times \frac{\overset{2}{\cancel{14}}}{21}$

Step 3: Cancel the 3 and 21: $\frac{\overset{1}{\cancel{3}}}{\underset{2}{\cancel{10}}} \times \frac{\overset{1}{\cancel{5}}}{\underset{1}{\cancel{7}}} \times \frac{\overset{2}{\cancel{14}}}{\underset{7}{\cancel{21}}}$

Step 4: Cancel the 2's: $\frac{\overset{1}{\cancel{3}}}{\underset{\underset{1}{2}}{\cancel{10}}} \times \frac{\overset{1}{\cancel{5}}}{\underset{1}{\cancel{7}}} \times \frac{\overset{\overset{1}{2}}{\cancel{14}}}{\underset{7}{\cancel{21}}}$

Step 5: Multiply the fractions: $\frac{\overset{1}{\cancel{3}}}{\underset{\underset{1}{2}}{\cancel{10}}} \times \frac{\overset{1}{\cancel{5}}}{\underset{1}{\cancel{7}}} \times \frac{\overset{\overset{1}{2}}{\cancel{14}}}{\underset{7}{\cancel{21}}} = \frac{1 \times 1 \times 1}{1 \times 1 \times 7} = \frac{1}{7}$

Thus: $\frac{3}{10} \times \frac{5}{7} \times \frac{14}{21} = \frac{1}{7}$

Note: The order in which the numbers are canceled is not important.

EXERCISES IN CANCELING FRACTIONS WHEN MULTIPLYING

(Answers are on pages 104–105.)

Multiply these fractions using the canceling method.

1) $\frac{2}{5} \times \frac{1}{2}$

2) $\frac{1}{3} \times \frac{3}{8}$

3) $\frac{7}{8} \times \frac{5}{14}$

4) $\frac{2}{3} \times \frac{3}{4}$

5) $\frac{5}{6} \times \frac{4}{5}$

6) $\frac{7}{9} \times \frac{3}{7}$

7) $\frac{3}{10} \times \frac{5}{9}$

8) $\frac{7}{11} \times \frac{33}{35}$

9) $\frac{5}{9} \times \frac{9}{10}$

10) $\frac{9}{16} \times \frac{4}{9}$

11) $\frac{3}{8} \times \frac{4}{15}$

12) $\frac{3}{10} \times \frac{5}{12}$

13) $\frac{3}{8} \times \frac{2}{5} \times \frac{2}{3}$

14) $\frac{4}{5} \times \frac{3}{4} \times \frac{5}{9}$

15) $\frac{11}{13} \times \frac{26}{33} \times \frac{3}{4}$

16) $\frac{5}{6} \times \frac{3}{10} \times \frac{3}{4}$

17) $\frac{10}{11} \times \frac{11}{15} \times \frac{1}{2}$

18) $\frac{2}{3} \times \frac{3}{4} \times \frac{4}{5} \times \frac{5}{6}$

MULTIPLYING WHOLE NUMBERS AND FRACTIONS

> To multiply a whole number times a fraction, convert the whole number to a fraction by placing the number over a denominator of one. Cancel when possible, and then multiply the fractions.

Example 7

Multiply $5 \times \frac{3}{5}$

Step 1: Convert 5 to a fraction: $\frac{5}{1} \times \frac{3}{5}$

Step 2: Cancel the 5's: $\frac{\overset{1}{\cancel{5}}}{1} \times \frac{3}{\underset{1}{\cancel{5}}}$

Step 3: Multiply the fractions: $\frac{\overset{1}{\cancel{5}}}{1} \times \frac{3}{\underset{1}{\cancel{5}}} = \frac{1 \times 3}{1 \times 1} = 3.$

Thus: $5 \times \frac{3}{5} = 3.$

Example 8

Multiply $\frac{2}{3} \times 12.$

Step 1: Convert 12 to a fraction: $\frac{2}{3} \times \frac{12}{1}$

Step 2: Cancel the 3 and 12: $\frac{2}{\underset{1}{\cancel{3}}} \times \frac{\overset{4}{\cancel{12}}}{1}$

Step 3: Multiply the fractions: $\frac{2}{\underset{1}{\cancel{3}}} \times \frac{\overset{4}{\cancel{12}}}{1} = \frac{2 \times 4}{1 \times 1} = 8.$

Thus: $\frac{2}{3} \times 12 = 8.$

EXERCISES IN MULTIPLYING WHOLE NUMBERS AND FRACTIONS

(Answers are on pages 105–106.)

Multiply these whole numbers and fractions. Cancel when possible.

1) $6 \times \frac{1}{2}$

2) $4 \times \frac{3}{8}$

3) $2 \times \frac{1}{8}$

4) $\frac{3}{5} \times 10$

5) $\frac{3}{4} \times 6$

6) $\frac{5}{7} \times 14$

7) $4 \times \frac{3}{4}$

8) $\frac{2}{3} \times 12$

MULTIPLYING MIXED NUMBERS

> To multiply mixed numbers, convert the mixed numbers to improper fractions. Cancel when possible, and then multiply the fractions.

Example 9

Multiply $1\frac{1}{2} \times \frac{1}{3}$

Step 1: Convert $1\frac{1}{2}$ to an improper fraction: $1\frac{1}{2} = \frac{3}{2}$

Step 2: Cancel the 3's: $\frac{\overset{1}{\cancel{3}}}{2} \times \frac{1}{\underset{1}{\cancel{3}}}$

Step 3: Multiply the fractions: $\frac{\overset{1}{\cancel{3}}}{2} \times \frac{1}{\underset{1}{\cancel{3}}} = \frac{1 \times 1}{2 \times 1} = \frac{1}{2}$

Thus: $1\frac{1}{2} \times \frac{1}{3} = \frac{1}{2}$

Example 10

Multiply $2\frac{1}{2} \times 1\frac{1}{4}$

Step 1: Convert the mixed numbers to improper fractions: $2\frac{1}{2} = \frac{5}{2}$ and $1\frac{1}{4} = \frac{5}{4}$

Step 2: Multiply the fractions. Turn the improper fraction into a mixed number and reduce the answer: $\frac{5}{2} \times \frac{5}{4} = \frac{25}{8} = 3\frac{1}{8}$

Thus: $2\frac{1}{2} \times 1\frac{1}{4} = 3\frac{1}{8}$

EXERCISES IN MULTIPLYING MIXED NUMBERS

(Answers are on pages 106–107.)

Multiply these mixed numbers.

1) $1\frac{3}{4} \times \frac{1}{2}$

2) $\frac{2}{3} \times 2\frac{1}{4}$

3) $1\frac{2}{3} \times \frac{1}{2}$

4) $\frac{2}{5} \times 1\frac{1}{4}$

5) $\frac{3}{5} \times 3\frac{1}{8}$

6) $4\frac{3}{8} \times 2$

7) $3 \times 2\frac{1}{3}$

8) $2\frac{2}{5} \times 3\frac{3}{4}$

9) $2\frac{2}{9} \times 2\frac{1}{10}$

10) $3\frac{3}{4} \times 1\frac{3}{5}$

11) $2\frac{2}{5} \times 4\frac{1}{6}$

12) $2\frac{2}{3} \times 1\frac{1}{8}$

13) $1\frac{1}{5} \times 2\frac{1}{2} \times 3\frac{3}{4}$

14) $2\frac{4}{5} \times \frac{4}{7} \times 3\frac{1}{2} \times \frac{5}{7}$

SOLVING MULTIPLICATION APPLICATIONS

> Multiplication application problems generally give information about one item and ask for information representing several of these items.
>
> The following key words may indicate the need to multiply: *product, times, of,* or *multiplied by.*
>
> For instance, if one shirt costs $5, how much would 3 shirts cost? To solve this, multiply the cost of one shirt ($5) by the number of shirts (3) to get the cost of those shirts ($15).

Example 11

A nurse's normal work week is $37\frac{1}{2}$ hr. This week the nurse worked $1\frac{1}{4}$ times as much. How many hours did the nurse work?

Multiply the hours in a normal work week times the fraction of time the nurse worked to find how many hours the nurse worked.

Step 1: Convert the mixed numbers to fractions: $37\frac{1}{2} = \frac{75}{2}$ and $1\frac{1}{4} = \frac{5}{4}$

Step 2: Multiply the fractions, and convert the answer to a mixed number.

$$\frac{75}{2} \times \frac{5}{4} = \frac{75 \times 5}{2 \times 4} = \frac{375}{8} = 46\frac{7}{8}$$

Thus, the nurse worked $46\frac{7}{8}$ hr.

Exercise 12

A bottle of medication contains 30 doses. There are $6\frac{3}{4}$ bottles on hand. How many doses are available?

Multiply the number of doses in a bottle (30) times the number of bottles on hand $\left(6\frac{3}{4}\right)$ to find out how many doses are available.

Step 1: Convert both numbers to improper fractions: $30 = \frac{30}{1}$ and $6\frac{3}{4} = \frac{27}{4}$

Step 2: Multiply the improper fractions, canceling where possible. Convert the answer to a mixed number.

$$\frac{\overset{15}{30}}{1} \times \frac{27}{\underset{2}{4}} = \frac{15 \times 27}{1 \times 2} = \frac{405}{2} = 202\frac{1}{2}$$

Thus, there are 202 doses available. The $\frac{1}{2}$ dose would not be given.

EXERCISES IN SOLVING MULTIPLICATION APPLICATIONS

(*Answers are on pages 107–108.*)

Solve these application problems using multiplication.

1) One tablet contains $2\frac{1}{2}$ grams of medication. If a patient was given $1\frac{1}{2}$ tablets, how many grams of medication did the patient receive?

2) One tablet contains 400 mg of medication. A patient was given $2\frac{1}{2}$ tablets. How many mg of medication did the patient received?

3) One tablet contains 600 mg of medication. A patient was given $1\frac{1}{2}$ tablets, how many mg of medication did the patient receive?

4) Each bottle contains $5\frac{1}{3}$ oz of hand sanitizer. How many oz of sanitizer are there in $4\frac{1}{2}$ bottles?

5) A resident is given $6\frac{2}{3}$ oz of orange juice every morning for 15 days. How many oz of orange juice was the patient given in this time period?

6) A bag contains $6\frac{1}{8}$ oz of saline solution. How much saline is present in 8 bags?

7) A dietician is preparing canned soup for a meal at the nursing facility. One can holds $8\frac{4}{5}$ oz. How many oz are in $\frac{5}{8}$ of a can?

8) The average dosage of a particular medicine is $\frac{2}{3}$ oz. If a resident was given 6 doses, how much medication was the resident given?

EXERCISES IN SOLVING MIXED APPLICATIONS

(Answers are on pages 109–110.)

Solve these application problems using addition, subtraction, and multiplication.

1) The average dose of a medicine is $1\frac{1}{2}$ oz. If a patient was given $\frac{2}{3}$ of a dose, how many oz of medication did the patient receive?

2) If $2\frac{1}{4}$ oz are removed from a bottle of cough syrup containing 6 oz, how many oz remain?

3) A resident was given a 16 oz container of water to drink throughout the day. If the resident drank $\frac{7}{8}$ of the container, how many oz did the resident drink?

4)   One drawer of a file cabinet containing old medical records is about $\frac{2}{3}$ full. Another drawer is about $\frac{1}{4}$ full. Can the records be combined in one drawer?

5)   If a resident eats $\frac{2}{3}$ of a $\frac{3}{4}$ oz candy bar, how many oz of candy is left?

SECTION TEST: MULTIPLICATION OF FRACTIONS

(Answers are on pages 110–112.)

Multiply these fractions. Cancel when possible.

1) $\frac{2}{3} \times \frac{1}{5}$

2) $\frac{1}{3} \times \frac{5}{7}$

3) $\frac{3}{5} \times \frac{3}{4}$

4) $\frac{3}{4} \times \frac{2}{5}$

5) $\frac{2}{3} \times \frac{3}{8}$

6) $\frac{5}{14} \times \frac{7}{15}$

7) $\frac{1}{2} \times \frac{3}{5} \times \frac{10}{21}$

8) $\frac{3}{5} \times \frac{5}{8} \times \frac{2}{3}$

9) $\frac{7}{8} \times \frac{2}{3} \times \frac{2}{7}$

10) $3 \times \frac{2}{3}$

11) $\frac{3}{8} \times 2$

12) $2 \times \frac{4}{5}$

13) $\frac{2}{3} \times 18$

14) $1\frac{1}{3} \times \frac{3}{8}$

15) $\frac{5}{8} \times 1\frac{3}{5}$

16) $1\frac{1}{2} \times 1\frac{1}{3}$

17) $3\frac{3}{4} \times 2\frac{2}{5}$

18) $4\frac{1}{5} \times 1\frac{1}{7}$

19) $4\frac{4}{5} \times 1\frac{2}{3}$

20) $2\frac{2}{3} \times 1\frac{1}{8}$

21) $1\frac{4}{5} \times 1\frac{2}{3} \times 1\frac{1}{4}$

22) One tablet contains 300 mg of medication. A patient was given $2\frac{1}{2}$ tablets. How much medication did the patient receive?

23) Each bottle holds $4\frac{1}{2}$ oz of cough syrup. How many oz of cough syrup are on hand if there are $5\frac{1}{3}$ bottles?

24) A resident drinks $5\frac{3}{4}$ oz of tomato juice every morning for 4 days. How many oz of tomato juice did the resident drink?

25) A bag contains $6\frac{2}{3}$ oz of saline solution. How many oz of saline solution are present in 6 bags?

26) The average dosage of a particular medicine is $\frac{3}{4}$ oz. If a resident was given 8 doses, how many oz of medication was the resident given?

ANSWERS TO EXERCISES IN MULTIPLYING FRACTIONS

(*Exercises are on page 87.*)

1) $\dfrac{3}{5} \times \dfrac{1}{4} = \dfrac{3 \times 1}{5 \times 4} = \dfrac{3}{20}$

2) $\dfrac{5}{9} \times \dfrac{1}{2} = \dfrac{5 \times 1}{9 \times 2} = \dfrac{5}{18}$

3) $\dfrac{3}{5} \times \dfrac{6}{7} = \dfrac{3 \times 6}{5 \times 7} = \dfrac{18}{35}$

4) $\dfrac{3}{4} \times \dfrac{3}{5} = \dfrac{3 \times 3}{4 \times 5} = \dfrac{9}{20}$

5) $\dfrac{1}{2} \times \dfrac{2}{3} = \dfrac{1 \times 2}{2 \times 3} = \dfrac{2}{6} = \dfrac{1}{3}$

6) $\dfrac{5}{8} \times \dfrac{3}{4} = \dfrac{5 \times 3}{8 \times 4} = \dfrac{15}{32}$

7) $\dfrac{4}{5} \times \dfrac{1}{8} = \dfrac{4 \times 1}{5 \times 8} = \dfrac{4}{40} = \dfrac{1}{10}$

8) $\dfrac{3}{4} \times \dfrac{3}{4} = \dfrac{3 \times 3}{4 \times 4} = \dfrac{9}{16}$

9) $\dfrac{7}{8} \times \dfrac{5}{7} = \dfrac{7 \times 5}{8 \times 7} = \dfrac{35}{56} = \dfrac{5}{8}$

10) $\dfrac{1}{2} \times \dfrac{1}{4} \times \dfrac{3}{4} = \dfrac{1 \times 1 \times 3}{2 \times 4 \times 4} = \dfrac{3}{32}$

11) $\dfrac{1}{2} \times \dfrac{3}{4} \times \dfrac{3}{5} = \dfrac{1 \times 3 \times 3}{2 \times 4 \times 5} = \dfrac{9}{40}$

12) $\dfrac{1}{2} \times \dfrac{3}{5} \times \dfrac{1}{2} = \dfrac{1 \times 3 \times 1}{2 \times 5 \times 2} = \dfrac{3}{20}$

ANSWERS TO EXERCISES IN CANCELING FRACTIONS WHEN MULTIPLYING

(*Exercises are on page 90.*)

1) $\dfrac{\overset{1}{2}}{5} \times \dfrac{1}{\underset{1}{2}} = \dfrac{1 \times 1}{5 \times 1} = \dfrac{1}{5}$

2) $\dfrac{1}{\underset{1}{3}} \times \dfrac{\overset{1}{3}}{8} = \dfrac{1 \times 1}{1 \times 8} = \dfrac{1}{8}$

3) $\dfrac{\overset{1}{7}}{8} \times \dfrac{5}{\underset{2}{14}} = \dfrac{1 \times 5}{8 \times 2} = \dfrac{5}{16}$

4) $\dfrac{\overset{1}{2}}{\underset{1}{3}} \times \dfrac{\overset{1}{3}}{\underset{2}{4}} = \dfrac{1 \times 1}{1 \times 2} = \dfrac{1}{2}$

5) $\dfrac{\overset{1}{5}}{\underset{3}{6}} \times \dfrac{\overset{2}{4}}{\underset{1}{5}} = \dfrac{1 \times 2}{3 \times 1} = \dfrac{2}{3}$

6) $\dfrac{\overset{1}{7}}{\underset{3}{9}} \times \dfrac{\overset{1}{3}}{\underset{1}{7}} = \dfrac{1 \times 1}{3 \times 1} = \dfrac{1}{3}$

7) $\dfrac{\overset{1}{3}}{\underset{2}{10}} \times \dfrac{\overset{1}{5}}{\underset{3}{9}} = \dfrac{1 \times 1}{2 \times 3} = \dfrac{1}{6}$

8) $\dfrac{\overset{1}{7}}{\underset{1}{11}} \times \dfrac{\overset{3}{33}}{\underset{5}{35}} = \dfrac{1 \times 3}{1 \times 5} = \dfrac{3}{5}$

9) $\dfrac{\overset{1}{5}}{\underset{1}{9}} \times \dfrac{\overset{1}{9}}{\underset{2}{10}} = \dfrac{1 \times 1}{1 \times 2} = \dfrac{1}{2}$

10) $\dfrac{\overset{1}{9}}{\underset{4}{16}} \times \dfrac{\overset{1}{4}}{\underset{1}{9}} = \dfrac{1 \times 1}{4 \times 1} = \dfrac{1}{4}$

11) $\dfrac{\overset{1}{\cancel{3}}}{\underset{2}{\cancel{8}}} \times \dfrac{\overset{1}{\cancel{4}}}{\underset{5}{\cancel{15}}} = \dfrac{1 \times 1}{2 \times 5} = \dfrac{1}{10}$

12) $\dfrac{\overset{1}{\cancel{3}}}{\underset{2}{\cancel{10}}} \times \dfrac{\overset{1}{\cancel{5}}}{\underset{4}{\cancel{12}}} = \dfrac{1 \times 1}{2 \times 4} = \dfrac{1}{8}$

13) $\dfrac{\overset{1}{\cancel{3}}}{\underset{\underset{2}{4}}{\cancel{8}}} \times \dfrac{\overset{1}{\cancel{2}}}{5} \times \dfrac{\overset{1}{\cancel{2}}}{\underset{1}{\cancel{3}}} = \dfrac{1 \times 1 \times 1}{2 \times 5 \times 1} = \dfrac{1}{10}$

14) $\dfrac{\overset{1}{\cancel{4}}}{\underset{1}{\cancel{5}}} \times \dfrac{\overset{1}{\cancel{3}}}{\underset{1}{\cancel{4}}} \times \dfrac{\overset{1}{\cancel{5}}}{\underset{3}{\cancel{9}}} = \dfrac{1 \times 1 \times 1}{1 \times 1 \times 3} = \dfrac{1}{3}$

15) $\dfrac{\overset{1}{\cancel{11}}}{\underset{1}{\cancel{13}}} \times \dfrac{\overset{\overset{1}{\cancel{2}}}{\cancel{26}}}{\underset{\underset{1}{3}}{\cancel{33}}} \times \dfrac{\overset{1}{\cancel{3}}}{\underset{2}{\cancel{4}}} = \dfrac{1 \times 1 \times 1}{1 \times 1 \times 2} = \dfrac{1}{2}$

16) $\dfrac{\overset{1}{\cancel{5}}}{\underset{2}{\cancel{6}}} \times \dfrac{\overset{1}{\cancel{3}}}{\underset{2}{\cancel{10}}} \times \dfrac{3}{4} = \dfrac{1 \times 1 \times 3}{2 \times 2 \times 4} = \dfrac{3}{16}$

17) $\dfrac{\overset{\overset{1}{\cancel{2}}}{\cancel{10}}}{\underset{1}{\cancel{11}}} \times \dfrac{\overset{1}{\cancel{11}}}{\underset{3}{\cancel{15}}} \times \dfrac{1}{\underset{1}{\cancel{2}}} = \dfrac{1 \times 1 \times 1}{1 \times 3 \times 1} = \dfrac{1}{3}$

18) $\dfrac{\overset{1}{\cancel{2}}}{\underset{1}{\cancel{3}}} \times \dfrac{\overset{1}{\cancel{3}}}{\underset{1}{\cancel{4}}} \times \dfrac{\overset{1}{\cancel{4}}}{\underset{1}{\cancel{5}}} \times \dfrac{\overset{1}{\cancel{5}}}{\underset{3}{\cancel{6}}} = \dfrac{1 \times 1 \times 1 \times 1}{1 \times 1 \times 1 \times 3} = \dfrac{1}{3}$

ANSWERS TO EXERCISES IN MULTIPLYING WHOLE NUMBERS AND FRACTIONS

(*Exercises are on page 92.*)

1) $6 \times \dfrac{1}{2} = \dfrac{\overset{3}{\cancel{6}}}{1} \times \dfrac{1}{\underset{1}{\cancel{2}}} = \dfrac{1 \times 3}{1 \times 1} = \dfrac{3}{1} = 3$

2) $4 \times \dfrac{3}{8} = \dfrac{\overset{1}{\cancel{4}}}{1} \times \dfrac{3}{\underset{2}{\cancel{8}}} = \dfrac{1 \times 3}{1 \times 2} = \dfrac{3}{2} = 1\dfrac{1}{2}$

3) $2 \times \dfrac{1}{8} = \dfrac{\overset{1}{\cancel{2}}}{1} \times \dfrac{1}{\underset{4}{\cancel{8}}} = \dfrac{1 \times 1}{1 \times 4} = \dfrac{1}{4}$

4) $\dfrac{3}{5} \times 10 = \dfrac{3}{\underset{1}{\cancel{5}}} \times \dfrac{\overset{2}{\cancel{10}}}{1} = \dfrac{3 \times 2}{1 \times 1} = \dfrac{6}{1} = 6$

5) $\dfrac{3}{4} \times 6 = \dfrac{3}{\underset{2}{\cancel{4}}} \times \dfrac{\overset{3}{\cancel{6}}}{1} = \dfrac{3 \times 3}{2 \times 1} = \dfrac{9}{2} = 4\dfrac{1}{2}$

6) $\dfrac{5}{7} \times 14 = \dfrac{5}{\underset{1}{\cancel{7}}} \times \dfrac{\overset{2}{\cancel{14}}}{1} = \dfrac{5 \times 2}{1 \times 1} = \dfrac{10}{1} = 10$

7) $4 \times \frac{3}{4} = \frac{\overset{1}{\cancel{4}}}{1} \times \frac{3}{\underset{1}{\cancel{4}}} = \frac{1 \times 3}{1 \times 1} = \frac{3}{1} = 3$

8) $\frac{2}{3} \times 12 = \frac{2}{\underset{1}{\cancel{3}}} \times \frac{\overset{4}{\cancel{12}}}{1} = \frac{2 \times 4}{1 \times 1} = \frac{8}{1} = 8$

ANSWERS TO EXERCISES IN MULTIPLYING MIXED NUMBERS

(Exercises are on pages 94–95.)

1) $1\frac{3}{4} \times \frac{1}{2} = \frac{7}{4} \times \frac{1}{2} = \frac{7 \times 1}{4 \times 2} = \frac{7}{8}$

2) $\frac{2}{3} \times 2\frac{1}{4} = \frac{2}{3} \times \frac{9}{4} = \frac{\overset{1}{\cancel{2}}}{\underset{1}{\cancel{3}}} \times \frac{\overset{3}{\cancel{9}}}{\underset{2}{\cancel{4}}} = \frac{1 \times 3}{1 \times 2} = \frac{3}{2} = 1\frac{1}{2}$

3) $1\frac{2}{3} \times \frac{1}{2} = \frac{5}{3} \times \frac{1}{2} = \frac{5 \times 1}{3 \times 2} = \frac{5}{6}$

4) $\frac{2}{5} \times 1\frac{1}{4} = \frac{2}{5} \times \frac{5}{4} = \frac{\overset{1}{\cancel{2}}}{\underset{1}{\cancel{5}}} \times \frac{\overset{1}{\cancel{5}}}{\underset{1}{\cancel{4}}} = \frac{1 \times 1}{1 \times 2} = \frac{1}{2}$

5) $\frac{3}{5} \times 3\frac{1}{8} = \frac{3}{5} \times \frac{25}{8} = \frac{3}{\underset{1}{\cancel{5}}} \times \frac{\overset{5}{\cancel{25}}}{8} = \frac{3 \times 5}{1 \times 8} = \frac{15}{8} = 1\frac{7}{8}$

6) $4\frac{3}{8} \times 2 = \frac{35}{8} \times \frac{2}{1} = \frac{35}{\underset{4}{\cancel{8}}} \times \frac{\overset{1}{\cancel{2}}}{1} = \frac{35 \times 1}{4 \times 1} = \frac{35}{4} = 8\frac{3}{4}$

7) $3 \times 2\frac{1}{3} = \frac{3}{1} \times \frac{7}{3} = \frac{\overset{1}{\cancel{3}}}{1} \times \frac{7}{\underset{1}{\cancel{3}}} = \frac{1 \times 7}{1 \times 1} = \frac{7}{1} = 7$

8) $2\frac{2}{5} \times 3\frac{3}{4} = \frac{12}{5} \times \frac{15}{4} = \frac{\overset{3}{\cancel{12}}}{\underset{1}{\cancel{5}}} \times \frac{\overset{3}{\cancel{15}}}{\underset{1}{\cancel{4}}} = \frac{3 \times 3}{1 \times 1} = \frac{9}{1} = 9$

9) $2\frac{2}{9} \times 2\frac{1}{10} = \frac{20}{9} \times \frac{21}{10} = \frac{\overset{2}{\cancel{20}}}{\underset{3}{\cancel{9}}} \times \frac{\overset{7}{\cancel{21}}}{\underset{1}{\cancel{10}}} = \frac{2 \times 7}{3 \times 1} = \frac{14}{3} = 4\frac{2}{3}$

10) $3\frac{3}{4} \times 1\frac{3}{5} = \frac{15}{4} \times \frac{8}{5} = \frac{\overset{3}{\cancel{15}}}{\underset{1}{\cancel{4}}} \times \frac{\overset{2}{\cancel{8}}}{\underset{1}{\cancel{5}}} = \frac{3 \times 2}{1 \times 1} = \frac{6}{1} = 6$

11) $2\frac{2}{5} \times 4\frac{1}{6} = \frac{12}{5} \times \frac{25}{6} = \frac{\overset{2}{\cancel{12}}}{\underset{1}{\cancel{5}}} \times \frac{\overset{5}{\cancel{25}}}{\underset{1}{\cancel{6}}} = \frac{2 \times 5}{1 \times 1} = \frac{10}{1} = 10$

12) $2\frac{2}{3} \times 1\frac{1}{8} = \frac{8}{3} \times \frac{9}{8} = \frac{\overset{1}{\cancel{8}}}{\underset{1}{\cancel{3}}} \times \frac{\overset{3}{\cancel{9}}}{\underset{1}{\cancel{8}}} = \frac{1 \times 3}{1 \times 1} = \frac{3}{1} = 3$

13) $1\frac{1}{5} \times 2\frac{1}{2} \times 3\frac{3}{4} = \frac{6}{5} \times \frac{5}{2} \times \frac{15}{4} = \frac{\overset{3}{\cancel{6}}}{\underset{1}{\cancel{5}}} \times \frac{\overset{1}{\cancel{5}}}{\underset{1}{\cancel{2}}} \times \frac{15}{4} = \frac{3 \times 1 \times 15}{1 \times 1 \times 4} = \frac{45}{4} = 11\frac{1}{4}$

14) $2\frac{4}{5} \times \frac{4}{7} \times 3\frac{1}{2} \times \frac{5}{7} = \frac{14}{5} \times \frac{4}{7} \times \frac{7}{2} \times \frac{5}{7} = \frac{\overset{2}{\cancel{14}}}{\underset{1}{\cancel{5}}} \times \frac{\overset{2}{\cancel{4}}}{\underset{1}{\cancel{7}}} \times \frac{\overset{1}{\cancel{7}}}{\underset{1}{\cancel{2}}} \times \frac{\overset{1}{\cancel{5}}}{\underset{1}{\cancel{7}}} = \frac{2 \times 2 \times 1 \times 1}{1 \times 1 \times 1 \times 1} = \frac{4}{1} = 4$

ANSWERS TO EXERCISES IN SOLVING MULTIPLICATION APPLICATIONS

(*Exercises are on pages 97–98.*)

1) Multiply the $2\frac{1}{2}$ grams of medication in one tablet times the $1\frac{1}{2}$ tablets given to find how many grams of medication the patient received.

$2\frac{1}{2} \times 1\frac{1}{2} = \frac{5}{2} \times \frac{3}{2} = \frac{5 \times 3}{2 \times 2} = \frac{15}{4} = 3\frac{3}{4}$

The patient received $3\frac{3}{4}$ grams of medication.

2) Multiply the 400 mg of medication in 1 tablet times the $2\frac{1}{2}$ tablets given to find how much medication the patient received.

$400 \times 2\frac{1}{2} = \frac{\overset{200}{\cancel{400}}}{1} \times \frac{5}{\underset{1}{\cancel{2}}} = \frac{200 \times 5}{1 \times 1} = \frac{1000}{1} = 1000$

The patient received 1000 mg of medication.

3) Multiply the 600 mg of medication in 1 tablet times the $1\frac{1}{2}$ tablets given to find how much medication the patient received.

$600 \times 1\frac{1}{2} = \frac{\overset{300}{\cancel{600}}}{1} \times \frac{3}{\underset{1}{\cancel{2}}} = \frac{300 \times 3}{1 \times 1} = \frac{900}{1} = 900$

The patient received 900 mg of medication.

4) Multiply the $5\frac{1}{3}$ oz of hand sanitizer each bottle contains times the $4\frac{1}{2}$ bottles to find how many oz of hand sanitizer there are.

$$4\frac{1}{2} \times 5\frac{1}{3} = \frac{\overset{3}{\cancel{9}}}{\underset{1}{\cancel{2}}} \times \frac{\overset{8}{\cancel{16}}}{\underset{1}{\cancel{3}}} = \frac{3 \times 8}{1 \times 1} = \frac{24}{1} = 24$$

There are 24 oz of hand sanitizer in $4\frac{1}{2}$ bottles.

5) Multiply the $6\frac{2}{3}$ oz of orange juice the resident is given times 15 days to find how many oz of orange juice the patient was given in this time period.

$$6\frac{2}{3} \times 15 = \frac{20}{\underset{1}{\cancel{3}}} \times \frac{\overset{5}{\cancel{15}}}{1} = \frac{20 \times 5}{1 \times 1} = \frac{100}{1} = 100$$

The resident was given 100 oz of orange juice in 15 days.

6) Multiply the $6\frac{1}{8}$ oz of saline solution in 1 bag times 8 bags to find how much saline is present.

$$6\frac{1}{8} \times 8 = \frac{49}{\underset{1}{\cancel{8}}} \times \frac{\overset{1}{\cancel{8}}}{1} = \frac{49}{1} = 49$$

There are 49 oz of saline solution in the 8 bags.

7) Multiply the $8\frac{4}{5}$ oz of soup in 1 can times $\frac{5}{8}$ of a can to find how many oz of soup this is.

$$8\frac{4}{5} \times \frac{5}{8} = \frac{\overset{11}{\cancel{44}}}{\underset{1}{\cancel{5}}} \times \frac{\overset{1}{\cancel{5}}}{\underset{2}{\cancel{8}}} = \frac{11 \times 1}{1 \times 2} = \frac{11}{2} = 5\frac{1}{2}$$

There are $5\frac{1}{2}$ oz of soup in $\frac{5}{8}$ of a can.

8) Multiply the $\frac{2}{3}$ oz of an average dosage of medicine times the 6 doses to find how much medication was given to the resident.

$$\frac{2}{3} \times 6 = \frac{2}{\underset{1}{\cancel{3}}} \times \frac{\overset{2}{\cancel{6}}}{1} = \frac{2 \times 2}{1 \times 1} = \frac{4}{1} = 4$$

The resident was given 4 oz of medication.

ANSWERS TO EXERCISES IN SOLVING MIXED APPLICATIONS

(*Exercises are on pages 99–100.*)

1) Multiply the $1\frac{1}{2}$ oz in an average dose of a medicine times the $\frac{2}{3}$ of a dose the patient was given to find how many oz of medicine the patient received.

$$1\frac{1}{2} \times \frac{2}{3} = \frac{\overset{1}{\cancel{3}}}{\underset{1}{\cancel{2}}} \times \frac{\overset{1}{\cancel{2}}}{\underset{1}{\cancel{3}}} = \frac{1 \times 1}{1 \times 1} = \frac{1}{1} = 1$$

The patient received 1 oz of medicine.

2) Subtract $2\frac{1}{4}$ oz from the original 6 oz to find how many oz remain.

$$6 \quad = 5\frac{4}{4}$$
$$-2\frac{1}{4} = 2\frac{1}{4}$$
$$\overline{\phantom{-2\frac{1}{4} = } 3\frac{3}{4}}$$

$3\frac{3}{4}$ oz of cough syrup remain in the bottle.

3) Multiply the 16 oz of water in the container times the $\frac{7}{8}$ of the container to find how many oz of water the resident drank.

$$16 \times \frac{7}{8} = \frac{\overset{2}{\cancel{16}}}{1} \times \frac{7}{\underset{1}{\cancel{8}}} = \frac{2 \times 7}{1 \times 1} = \frac{14}{1} = 14$$

The resident drank 14 oz of water.

4) Add the $\frac{2}{3}$ full drawer and the $\frac{1}{4}$ full drawer together.

$$\frac{2}{3} = \frac{8}{12}$$
$$+\frac{1}{4} = \frac{3}{12}$$
$$\overline{\phantom{+\frac{1}{4} = } \frac{11}{12}}$$

Because a $\frac{11}{12}$ full drawer is less than 1 full drawer, the records will fit in 1 drawer.

5) This is a multistep problem. Multiply the $\frac{2}{3}$ that the resident ate times the $\frac{3}{4}$ oz in the candy bar to find how many oz of candy the resident ate.

$$\overset{1}{\underset{1}{\frac{2}{3}}} \times \overset{1}{\underset{2}{\frac{3}{4}}} = \frac{1 \times 1}{1 \times 2} = \frac{1}{2}$$

The resident ate $\frac{1}{2}$ oz of candy.

Now, subtract $\frac{1}{2}$ oz of candy the resident ate from the $\frac{3}{4}$ oz in the candy bar to find how many oz of candy is left.

$$\begin{array}{r} \frac{3}{4} = \frac{3}{4} \\ -\frac{1}{2} = \frac{2}{4} \\ \hline \frac{1}{4} \end{array}$$

There is $\frac{1}{4}$ oz of candy left.

ANSWERS TO SECTION TEST: MULTIPLICATION OF FRACTIONS

(*Section Test is on pages 101–103.*)

1) $\frac{2}{3} \times \frac{1}{5} = \frac{2 \times 1}{3 \times 5} = \frac{2}{15}$

2) $\frac{1}{3} \times \frac{5}{7} = \frac{1 \times 5}{3 \times 7} = \frac{5}{21}$

3) $\frac{3}{5} \times \frac{3}{4} = \frac{3 \times 3}{5 \times 4} = \frac{9}{20}$

4) $\frac{3}{\underset{2}{4}} \times \overset{1}{\frac{2}{5}} = \frac{3 \times 1}{2 \times 5} = \frac{3}{10}$

5) $\overset{1}{\underset{1}{\frac{2}{3}}} \times \overset{1}{\underset{4}{\frac{3}{8}}} = \frac{1 \times 1}{1 \times 4} = \frac{1}{4}$

6) $\overset{1}{\underset{2}{\frac{5}{14}}} \times \overset{1}{\underset{3}{\frac{7}{15}}} = \frac{1 \times 1}{2 \times 3} = \frac{1}{6}$

7) $\underset{1}{\frac{1}{2}} \times \overset{1}{\underset{1}{\frac{3}{5}}} \times \overset{\overset{1}{2}}{\underset{7}{\frac{10}{21}}} = \frac{1 \times 1 \times 1}{1 \times 1 \times 7} = \frac{1}{7}$

8) $\overset{1}{\underset{1}{\frac{3}{5}}} \times \overset{1}{\underset{4}{\frac{5}{8}}} \times \overset{1}{\underset{1}{\frac{2}{3}}} = \frac{1 \times 1 \times 1}{1 \times 4 \times 1} = \frac{1}{4}$

9) $\overset{1}{\underset{\underset{2}{4}}{\frac{7}{8}}} \times \overset{1}{\underset{3}{\frac{2}{3}}} \times \overset{1}{\underset{1}{\frac{2}{7}}} = \frac{1 \times 1 \times 1}{2 \times 3 \times 1} = \frac{1}{6}$

10) $3 \times \frac{2}{3} = \frac{3}{1} \times \frac{2}{\underset{1}{3}} = \frac{1 \times 2}{1 \times 1} = \frac{2}{1} = 2$

11) $\dfrac{3}{8} \times 2 = \dfrac{3}{\overset{}{\underset{4}{8}}} \times \dfrac{\overset{1}{2}}{1} = \dfrac{3 \times 1}{4 \times 1} = \dfrac{3}{4}$

12) $2 \times \dfrac{4}{5} = \dfrac{2}{1} \times \dfrac{4}{5} = \dfrac{2 \times 4}{1 \times 5} = \dfrac{8}{5} = 1\dfrac{3}{5}$

13) $\dfrac{2}{3} \times 18 = \dfrac{2}{\underset{1}{3}} \times \dfrac{\overset{6}{18}}{1} = \dfrac{2 \times 6}{1 \times 1} = \dfrac{12}{1} = 12$

14) $1\dfrac{1}{3} \times \dfrac{3}{8} = \dfrac{\overset{1}{4}}{\underset{1}{3}} \times \dfrac{\overset{1}{3}}{\underset{2}{8}} = \dfrac{1 \times 1}{1 \times 2} = \dfrac{1}{2}$

15) $\dfrac{5}{8} \times 1\dfrac{3}{5} = \dfrac{\overset{1}{5}}{\underset{1}{8}} \times \dfrac{\overset{1}{8}}{\underset{1}{5}} = \dfrac{1 \times 1}{1 \times 1} = \dfrac{1}{1} = 1$

16) $1\dfrac{1}{2} \times 1\dfrac{1}{3} = \dfrac{\overset{1}{3}}{\underset{1}{2}} \times \dfrac{\overset{2}{4}}{\underset{1}{3}} = \dfrac{1 \times 2}{1 \times 1} = \dfrac{2}{1} = 2$

17) $3\dfrac{3}{4} \times 2\dfrac{2}{5} = \dfrac{\overset{3}{15}}{\underset{1}{4}} \times \dfrac{\overset{3}{12}}{\underset{1}{5}} = \dfrac{3 \times 3}{1 \times 1} = \dfrac{9}{1} = 9$

18) $4\dfrac{1}{5} \times 1\dfrac{1}{7} = \dfrac{21}{5} \times \dfrac{\overset{3}{21}}{\underset{1}{7}} \cdot \dfrac{8}{7} = \dfrac{3 \times 8}{5 \times 1} = \dfrac{24}{5} = 4\dfrac{4}{5}$

19) $4\dfrac{4}{5} \times 1\dfrac{2}{3} = \dfrac{\overset{8}{24}}{\underset{1}{5}} \times \dfrac{\overset{1}{5}}{\underset{1}{3}} = \dfrac{8 \times 1}{1 \times 1} = \dfrac{8}{1} = 8$

20) $2\dfrac{2}{3} \times 1\dfrac{1}{8} = \dfrac{\overset{1}{8}}{\underset{1}{3}} \times \dfrac{\overset{3}{9}}{\underset{1}{8}} = \dfrac{1 \times 3}{1 \times 1} = \dfrac{3}{1} = 3$

21) $1\dfrac{4}{5} \times 1\dfrac{2}{3} \times 1\dfrac{1}{4} = \dfrac{\overset{3}{9}}{\underset{1}{5}} \times \dfrac{\overset{1}{5}}{\underset{1}{3}} \times \dfrac{5}{4} = \dfrac{3 \times 1 \times 5}{1 \times 1 \times 4} = \dfrac{15}{4} = 3\dfrac{3}{4}$

22) Multiply the 300 mg of medication in one tablet times the $2\dfrac{1}{2}$ tablets the patient was given to find how much medication the patient received.

$$300 \times 2\dfrac{1}{2} = \dfrac{\overset{150}{300}}{1} \times \dfrac{5}{\underset{1}{2}} = \dfrac{150 \times 5}{1 \times 1} = \dfrac{750}{1} = 750$$

The patient received 750 mg of medication.

23) Multiply the $4\frac{1}{2}$ oz of cough syrup in 1 bottle times $5\frac{1}{3}$ bottles to find how many oz of cough syrup are on hand.

$$4\frac{1}{2} \times 5\frac{1}{3} = \frac{\overset{3}{\cancel{9}}}{\underset{1}{\cancel{2}}} \times \frac{\overset{8}{\cancel{16}}}{\underset{1}{\cancel{3}}} = \frac{3 \times 8}{1 \times 1} = \frac{24}{1} = 24$$

There are 24 oz of cough syrup on hand.

24) Multiply the $5\frac{3}{4}$ oz of tomato juice the resident drinks every morning times 4 days to find how many oz of tomato juice the resident drank.

$$5\frac{3}{4} \times 4 = \frac{23}{\underset{1}{\cancel{4}}} \times \frac{\overset{1}{\cancel{4}}}{1} = \frac{23 \times 1}{1 \times 1} = \frac{23}{1} = 23$$

The resident drank 23 oz of tomato juice in 4 days.

25) Multiply the $6\frac{2}{3}$ oz of saline solution in 1 bag times 6 bags to find how many oz of saline solution are present.

$$6\frac{2}{3} \times 6 = \frac{20}{\underset{1}{\cancel{3}}} \times \frac{\overset{2}{\cancel{6}}}{1} = \frac{20 \times 2}{1 \times 1} = \frac{40}{1} = 40$$

There are 40 oz of saline solution present.

26) Multiply the $\frac{3}{4}$ oz average dosage of medicine times the 8 doses to find how many oz of medication were given to the resident.

$$\frac{3}{4} \times 8 = \frac{3}{\underset{1}{\cancel{4}}} \times \frac{\overset{2}{\cancel{8}}}{1} = \frac{3 \times 2}{1 \times 1} = \frac{6}{1} = 6$$

The resident was given 6 oz of medication.

Division of Fractions

OBJECTIVES

Upon completion of this section, you should be able to:

1) Create the reciprocal of a fraction.
2) Create the reciprocal of a whole number.
3) Rewrite a division problem as multiplication by a reciprocal.
4) Divide a fraction by a fraction.
5) Divide a whole number by a fraction.
6) Divide a fraction by a whole number.
7) Divide mixed numbers.

CREATING RECIPROCALS OF FRACTIONS

A **reciprocal** of a fraction is its inverse. The numerator in the fraction is used as the denominator of the reciprocal, and the denominator of the fraction is used as the numerator of the reciprocal. The reciprocal of $\frac{2}{3}$ is $\frac{3}{2}$

A fraction multiplied by its reciprocal equals 1. $\frac{\overset{1}{\cancel{2}}}{\underset{1}{\cancel{3}}} \times \frac{\overset{1}{\cancel{3}}}{\underset{1}{\cancel{2}}} = \frac{1}{1} = 1$

Example 1

1a) *What is the reciprocal of $\frac{3}{4}$?*

The reciprocal of $\frac{3}{4}$ is $\frac{4}{3}$

1b) *What is the reciprocal of $\frac{5}{8}$?*

The reciprocal of $\frac{5}{8}$ is $\frac{8}{5}$

Example 2

2a) *Multiply $\frac{3}{4}$ by its reciprocal.*

$$\frac{\overset{1}{\cancel{3}}}{\underset{1}{\cancel{4}}}\times\frac{\overset{1}{\cancel{4}}}{\underset{1}{\cancel{3}}}=\frac{1}{1}=1$$

2b) *Multiply $\frac{5}{8}$ by its reciprocal.*

$$\frac{\overset{1}{\cancel{5}}}{\underset{1}{\cancel{8}}}\times\frac{\overset{1}{\cancel{8}}}{\underset{1}{\cancel{5}}}=\frac{1}{1}=1$$

CREATING RECIPROCALS OF WHOLE NUMBERS

To find the reciprocal of a whole number, turn the whole number into a fraction and then create its reciprocal. To find the reciprocal of 2, turn 2 into the fraction $\frac{2}{1}$. The reciprocal of $\frac{2}{1}$ is $\frac{1}{2}$

Example 3

3a) *What is the reciprocal of 5?*

$5=\frac{5}{1}$, so the reciprocal of $\frac{5}{1}$ is $\frac{1}{5}$

3b) *What is the reciprocal of 8?*

$8=\frac{8}{1}$, so the reciprocal of $\frac{8}{1}$ is $\frac{1}{8}$

EXERCISES IN RECIPROCALS OF FRACTIONS AND WHOLE NUMBERS

(Answers are on page 141.)

What are the reciprocals of these fractions?

1) $\frac{3}{4}$

2) $\frac{2}{5}$

3) $\frac{7}{8}$

4) $\frac{4}{9}$

5) $\frac{1}{10}$

6) $\frac{5}{7}$

7) $\frac{11}{12}$

8) $\frac{9}{16}$

9) $\frac{13}{16}$

What are the reciprocals of these whole numbers?

10) 3

11) 5

12) 7

13) 12

14) 100

15) 1

REWRITING A DIVISION PROBLEM AS MULTIPLICATION BY A RECIPROCAL

> Dividing by a number will give the same answer as multiplying by the number's reciprocal. Example: $6 \div 2 = 3$. Because the reciprocal of 2 is $\frac{1}{2}$, multiplying 6 times $\frac{1}{2}$ will give the same
>
> answer: $6 \times \frac{1}{2} = \frac{\overset{3}{\cancel{6}}}{1} \times \frac{1}{\underset{1}{\cancel{2}}} = \frac{3}{1} = 3$
>
> Because of this, when working with fractions, instead of dividing, we multiply by the reciprocal of the divisor.
>
> To rewrite a division problem as multiplication by a reciprocal, do these steps.
>
> Step 1:   Leave the first number as it is.
>
> Step 2:   Change the division sign to the multiplication sign.
>
> Step 3:   Find the reciprocal of the divisor (the number after the division sign). Change the divisor to its reciprocal.

Example 4

Rewrite these division problems as multiplication problems using reciprocals.

4a) $12 \div 4$

   $12 \div 4$ is the same as $\frac{12}{1} \times \frac{1}{4}$

4b) $2 \div \frac{1}{4}$

   $2 \div \frac{1}{4}$ is the same as $\frac{2}{1} \times \frac{4}{1}$

EXERCISES IN REWRITING A DIVISION PROBLEM AS MULTIPLICATION BY A RECIPROCAL

(Answers are on page 141.)

Rewrite these division problems as multiplication by a reciprocal. Do not solve the problems.

1) $\frac{1}{2} \div \frac{3}{4}$

2) $\frac{3}{5} \div \frac{4}{7}$

3) $\frac{5}{9} \div \frac{2}{7}$

4) $\frac{1}{3} \div \frac{2}{5}$

5) $\frac{7}{8} \div \frac{7}{8}$

6) $8 \div 4$

7) $5 \div 3$

8) $9 \div \frac{1}{3}$

9) $10 \div \frac{2}{5}$

10) $\frac{1}{2} \div 3$

11) $\frac{3}{8} \div 6$

12) $\frac{3}{4} \div 9$

DIVIDING A FRACTION BY A FRACTION

> Instead of dividing by a fraction, multiply by the reciprocal of the fraction. In other words, change the division sign to multiplication and multiply by the reciprocal of the divisor.

Example 5

Solve this division problem by changing it to a multiplication problem using the reciprocal of the divisor: $\frac{1}{3} \div \frac{1}{2}$

Step 1:   Find the reciprocal of the divisor.
The divisor is $\frac{1}{2}$, so the reciprocal is $\frac{2}{1}$

Step 2:   Rewrite the division problem as a multiplication problem using the reciprocal.
$\frac{1}{3} \div \frac{1}{2}$ becomes $\frac{1}{3} \times \frac{2}{1}$

Step 3:   Solve the problem.
$\frac{1}{3} \times \frac{2}{1} = \frac{2}{3}$

Thus: $\frac{1}{3} \div \frac{1}{2} = \frac{2}{3}$

Example 6

Solve this division problem by changing it to a multiplication problem using the reciprocal of the divisor: $\frac{3}{4} \div \frac{1}{2}$

Step 1:   Find the reciprocal of the divisor.
The divisor is $\frac{1}{2}$, so the reciprocal is $\frac{2}{1}$

Step 2:   Rewrite the division problem as a multiplication problem using the reciprocal.
$\frac{3}{4} \div \frac{1}{2}$ becomes $\frac{3}{4} \times \frac{2}{1}$

Step 3:   Solve the problem.
$\frac{3}{\overset{}{4}} \times \overset{1}{\underset{2}{\frac{2}{1}}} = \frac{3}{2} = 1\frac{1}{2}$

Thus: $\frac{3}{4} \div \frac{1}{2} = 1\frac{1}{2}$

Example 7

Solve this division problem by changing it to a multiplication problem using the reciprocal of the divisor: $\frac{3}{4} \div \frac{3}{8}$

Step 1: Find the reciprocal of the divisor.

The divisor is $\frac{3}{8}$, so the reciprocal is $\frac{8}{3}$

Step 2: Rewrite the division problem as a multiplication problem using the reciprocal.

$\frac{3}{4} \div \frac{3}{8}$ becomes $\frac{3}{4} \times \frac{8}{3}$

Step 3: Solve the problem.

$$\frac{\overset{1}{\cancel{3}}}{\underset{1}{\cancel{4}}} \times \frac{\overset{2}{\cancel{8}}}{\underset{1}{\cancel{3}}} = \frac{2}{1} = 2$$

Thus: $\frac{3}{4} \div \frac{3}{8} = 2$

EXERCISES IN DIVIDING A FRACTION BY A FRACTION

(Answers are on page 142.)

Solve these division problems by multiplying by the reciprocal.

1) $\frac{3}{4} \div \frac{1}{2}$

2) $\frac{3}{4} \div \frac{3}{4}$

3) $\frac{2}{5} \div \frac{1}{2}$

4) $\frac{1}{8} \div \frac{1}{3}$

5) $\frac{1}{5} \div \frac{3}{5}$

6) $\frac{7}{8} \div \frac{1}{8}$

7) $\frac{3}{5} \div \frac{2}{5}$

8) $\frac{1}{2} \div \frac{5}{8}$

9) $\frac{3}{8} \div \frac{1}{4}$

10) $\frac{1}{3} \div \frac{2}{3}$

11) $\frac{1}{4} \div \frac{4}{5}$

12) $\frac{3}{4} \div \frac{2}{3}$

DIVIDING A WHOLE NUMBER BY A FRACTION

To divide a whole number by a fraction, turn the whole number into its equivalent fraction. Next, multiply by the reciprocal of the divisor.

Example 8

Divide 6 by $\frac{1}{2}$

Step 1:   Turn the whole number into a fraction. $6 = \frac{6}{1}$

Step 2:   Find the reciprocal of the divisor $\frac{1}{2}$

The divisor is $\frac{1}{2}$, so the reciprocal is $\frac{2}{1}$

Step 3:   Change the division problem into multiplication by the reciprocal.

$\frac{6}{1} \div \frac{1}{2}$ becomes $\frac{6}{1} \times \frac{2}{1}$

Step 4:   Solve the problem.

$\frac{6}{1} \times \frac{2}{1} = \frac{6 \times 2}{1 \times 1} = \frac{12}{1} = 12$

Thus: $\frac{6}{1} \div \frac{1}{2} = 12$

Example 9

Divide 12 by $\frac{2}{3}$

Step 1:   Turn the whole number into a fraction. $12 = \frac{12}{1}$

Step 2:   Find the reciprocal of the divisor $\frac{2}{3}$

The divisor is $\frac{2}{3}$, so the reciprocal is $\frac{3}{2}$

Step 3:   Change the division problem into multiplication by the reciprocal.

$\frac{12}{1} \div \frac{2}{3}$ becomes $\frac{12}{1} \times \frac{3}{2}$

Step 4:   Solve the problem.

$\frac{\overset{6}{\cancel{12}}}{1} \times \frac{3}{\underset{1}{\cancel{2}}} = \frac{6 \times 3}{1 \times 1} = \frac{18}{1} = 18$

Thus: $12 \div \frac{2}{3} = 18$

EXERCISES IN DIVIDING A WHOLE NUMBER BY A FRACTION

(Answers are on pages 142–143.)

Solve these division problems by multiplying by the reciprocal.

1) $4 \div \frac{1}{2}$

2) $3 \div \frac{1}{3}$

3) $6 \div \frac{2}{3}$

4) $10 \div \frac{5}{8}$

5) $12 \div \frac{3}{4}$

6) $12 \div \frac{3}{8}$

7) $5 \div \frac{1}{2}$

8) $14 \div \frac{7}{8}$

9) $2 \div \frac{2}{3}$

10) $1 \div \frac{5}{8}$

11) $4 \div \frac{3}{8}$

12) $6 \div \frac{3}{4}$

DIVIDING A FRACTION BY A WHOLE NUMBER

> To divide a fraction by a whole number, turn the whole number into its equivalent fraction. Next, multiply by the reciprocal of that fraction.

Example 10

Divide $\frac{1}{2}$ by 6

Step 1: Turn the whole number into a fraction. $6 = \frac{6}{1}$

Step 2: Find the reciprocal of the divisor $\frac{6}{1}$

The divisor is $\frac{6}{1}$, so the reciprocal is $\frac{1}{6}$

Step 3: Change the division problem into multiplication by the reciprocal.
$\frac{1}{2} \div \frac{6}{1}$ becomes $\frac{1}{2} \times \frac{1}{6}$

Step 4: Solve the problem.

$$\frac{1}{2} \times \frac{1}{6} = \frac{1 \times 1}{2 \times 6} = \frac{1}{12}$$

Thus: $\frac{1}{2} \div \frac{6}{1} = \frac{1}{12}$

EXERCISES IN DIVIDING A FRACTION BY A WHOLE NUMBER

(Answers are on page 143.)

Solve these division problems by multiplying by the reciprocal.

1) $\frac{1}{4} \div 2$

2) $\frac{3}{5} \div 6$

3) $\frac{7}{8} \div 7$

4) $\frac{3}{4} \div 12$

5) $\frac{2}{3} \div 12$

6) $\frac{3}{8} \div 12$

7) $\frac{3}{4} \div 2$

8) $\frac{1}{4} \div 4$

9) $\frac{5}{8} \div 2$

10) $\frac{3}{5} \div 3$

11) $\frac{7}{8} \div 14$

12) $\frac{2}{3} \div 8$

DIVIDING A MIXED NUMBER BY A WHOLE NUMBER

> To divide a mixed number by a whole number, follow these steps.
>
> Step 1: Turn the mixed number into an improper fraction.
>
> Step 2: Turn the whole number into a fraction.
>
> Step 3: Change the division problem into multiplication by the reciprocal.

Example 11

Divide $1\frac{1}{2}$ by 6

Step 1: Turn the mixed number into a fraction. $1\frac{1}{2} = \frac{3}{2}$

Step 2: Find the reciprocal of the divisor 6

The divisor is $\frac{6}{1}$, so the reciprocal is $\frac{1}{6}$

Step 3: Change the division problem into multiplication by the reciprocal.

$\frac{3}{2} \div \frac{6}{1}$ becomes $\frac{3}{2} \times \frac{1}{6}$

Step 4: Solve the problem.

$\frac{\overset{1}{\cancel{3}}}{2} \times \frac{1}{\underset{2}{\cancel{6}}} = \frac{1 \times 1}{2 \times 2} = \frac{1}{4}$

Thus: $1\frac{1}{2} \div 6 = \frac{1}{4}$

EXERCISES IN DIVIDING A MIXED NUMBER BY A WHOLE NUMBER

(Answers are on pages 143–144.)

Solve these division problems by multiplying by the reciprocal.

1) $1\frac{1}{2} \div 2$

2) $2\frac{2}{3} \div 4$

3) $1\frac{3}{5} \div 8$

4) $1\frac{1}{3} \div 8$

5) $1\frac{7}{8} \div 5$

6) $1\frac{1}{2} \div 5$

7) $2\frac{2}{3} \div 8$

8) $1\frac{3}{5} \div 4$

9) $5\frac{2}{5} \div 9$

10) $1\frac{1}{2} \div 9$

11) $2\frac{3}{4} \div 11$

12) $2\frac{2}{3} \div 12$

DIVIDING A MIXED NUMBER BY A FRACTION

> To divide a mixed number by a fraction, turn the mixed number into an improper fraction. Next, multiply by the reciprocal of the divisor.

Example 12

Divide $1\frac{1}{2}$ *by* $\frac{3}{4}$

Step 1:   Turn the mixed number into a fraction. $1\frac{1}{2} = \frac{3}{2}$

Step 2:   Find the reciprocal of the divisor $\frac{3}{4}$

        The divisor is $\frac{3}{4}$, so the reciprocal is $\frac{4}{3}$

Step 3:   Change the division problem into multiplication by the reciprocal.
$\frac{3}{2} \div \frac{3}{4}$ becomes $\frac{3}{2} \times \frac{4}{3}$

Step 4:   Solve the problem.
$$\frac{\overset{1}{\cancel{3}}}{\underset{1}{\cancel{2}}} \times \frac{\overset{2}{\cancel{4}}}{\underset{1}{\cancel{3}}} = \frac{1 \times 2}{1 \times 1} = \frac{2}{1} = 2$$

Thus: $1\frac{1}{2} \div \frac{3}{4} = 2$

EXERCISES IN DIVIDING A MIXED NUMBER BY A FRACTION

(Answers are on page 144.)

Solve these division problems by multiplying by the reciprocal.

1) $1\frac{1}{2} \div \frac{1}{3}$

2) $1\frac{3}{4} \div \frac{1}{2}$

3) $1\frac{1}{2} \div \frac{3}{4}$

4) $1\frac{1}{4} \div \frac{3}{8}$

5) $1\frac{1}{2} \div \frac{3}{8}$

6) $2\frac{3}{4} \div \frac{2}{5}$

7) $2\frac{3}{4} \div \frac{1}{2}$

8) $2\frac{2}{3} \div \frac{4}{5}$

9) $2\frac{5}{8} \div \frac{7}{8}$

10) $3\frac{1}{2} \div 1\frac{2}{5}$

11) $3\frac{2}{3} \div 2\frac{1}{5}$

12) $2\frac{2}{5} \div 3\frac{1}{3}$

DIVIDING A FRACTION BY A MIXED NUMBER

> To divide a fraction by a mixed number, turn the mixed number into an improper fraction. Next, multiply by the reciprocal of the divisor.

Example 13

Divide $\frac{3}{8}$ by $1\frac{1}{2}$

Step 1: Turn the mixed number into a fraction. $1\frac{1}{2} = \frac{3}{2}$

Step 2: Find the reciprocal of the divisor $\frac{3}{2}$

   The divisor is $\frac{3}{2}$, so the reciprocal is $\frac{2}{3}$

Step 3: Change the division problem into multiplication by the reciprocal.
   $\frac{3}{8} \div \frac{3}{2}$ becomes $\frac{3}{8} \times \frac{2}{3}$

Step 4: Solve the problem.

$$\frac{\overset{1}{\cancel{3}}}{\underset{4}{\cancel{8}}} \times \frac{\overset{1}{\cancel{2}}}{\underset{1}{\cancel{3}}} = \frac{1 \times 1}{4 \times 1} = \frac{1}{4}$$

Thus: $\frac{3}{8} \div 1\frac{1}{2} = \frac{1}{4}$

EXERCISES IN DIVIDING A FRACTION BY A MIXED NUMBER

(Answers are on page 145.)

Solve these division problems by multiplying by the reciprocal.

1) $\frac{1}{2} \div 1\frac{1}{2}$

2) $\frac{4}{5} \div 1\frac{1}{3}$

3) $\frac{3}{4} \div 1\frac{1}{2}$

4) $\frac{7}{8} \div 2\frac{5}{8}$

5) $\frac{3}{4} \div 1\frac{1}{4}$

6) $\frac{5}{8} \div 1\frac{2}{3}$

7) $\frac{3}{5} \div 1\frac{1}{2}$

8) $\frac{4}{5} \div 2\frac{2}{3}$

9) $\frac{5}{8} \div 1\frac{1}{4}$

10) $\frac{2}{3} \div 1\frac{2}{3}$

11) $\frac{3}{4} \div 1\frac{7}{8}$

12) $\frac{2}{5} \div 3\frac{3}{5}$

DIVIDING A MIXED NUMBER BY A MIXED NUMBER

> To divide a mixed number by a mixed number, turn both mixed numbers into improper fractions. Next, multiply by the reciprocal of the divisor.

Example 14

Divide $2\frac{1}{2}$ *by* $1\frac{1}{4}$

Step 1: Turn the mixed numbers into fractions.
$$2\frac{1}{2} = \frac{5}{2} \text{ and } 1\frac{1}{4} = \frac{5}{4}$$

Step 2: Find the reciprocal of the divisor $\frac{5}{4}$

The divisor is $\frac{5}{4}$, so the reciprocal is $\frac{4}{5}$

Step 3: Change the division problem into multiplication by the reciprocal.
$$\frac{5}{2} \div \frac{5}{4} \text{ becomes } \frac{5}{2} \times \frac{4}{5}$$

Step 4: Solve the problem.
$$2\frac{1}{2} \div 1\frac{1}{4} = \frac{5}{2} \div \frac{5}{4} = \frac{\overset{1}{\cancel{5}}}{\underset{1}{\cancel{2}}} \times \frac{\overset{2}{\cancel{4}}}{\underset{1}{\cancel{5}}} = \frac{1 \times 2}{1 \times 1} = \frac{2}{1} = 2$$

Thus: $2\frac{1}{2} \div 1\frac{1}{4} = 2$

EXERCISES IN DIVIDING A MIXED NUMBER BY A MIXED NUMBER

(Answers are on pages 145–146.)

Solve these division problems by multiplying by the reciprocal.

1) $1\frac{1}{8} \div 2\frac{1}{4}$

2) $1\frac{4}{5} \div 4\frac{1}{2}$

3) $1\frac{1}{4} \div 1\frac{7}{8}$

4) $2\frac{3}{4} \div 3\frac{3}{4}$

5) $4\frac{2}{3} \div 2\frac{1}{3}$

6) $1\frac{3}{7} \div 1\frac{2}{3}$

7) $2\frac{2}{3} \div 1\frac{7}{9}$

8) $5\frac{5}{8} \div 1\frac{1}{4}$

9) $1\frac{1}{4} \div 3\frac{1}{8}$

10) $2\frac{2}{5} \div 1\frac{1}{5}$

11) $2\frac{2}{3} \div 4\frac{4}{5}$

12) $4\frac{2}{3} \div 1\frac{2}{5}$

SOLVING DIVISION APPLICATIONS

> Division is used to take a larger quantity and divide it into an equal number of smaller parts.
>
> The following key words may indicate the need to divide: *per, average,* and *how much is each one.*
>
> For example, if $20 is being evenly split among 5 children, then $20 would be divided by 5 to get $4 as an answer. Thus, each child would get $4. To verify that this is correct, consider the reverse: if each child put his or her $4 together with the others, then they would have $20. ($4 × 5 = $20.)

Example 15

How many $2\frac{1}{2}$ oz doses of medication are there in a 20-oz bottle?

One way to solve this problem would be to physically pour out $2\frac{1}{2}$ oz doses from the 20-oz bottle and then count how many doses there are. An easier way would be to consider that the 20-oz bottle of medication has to be divided into $2\frac{1}{2}$ oz doses.

$$20 \div 2\frac{1}{2} = \frac{20}{1} \div \frac{5}{2} = \frac{\overset{4}{\cancel{20}}}{1} \times \frac{2}{\underset{1}{\cancel{5}}} = \frac{4 \times 2}{1 \times 1} = \frac{8}{1} = 8$$

The number of $2\frac{1}{2}$ oz doses of medication in a 20-oz bottle is 8.

EXERCISES IN SOLVING DIVISION APPLICATIONS

(Answers are on pages 146–148.)

Solve these fraction application problems.

1) Each patient in a nursing facility requires about $\frac{1}{3}$ hr for daily grooming by an attendant. How many patients can the attendant groom in 3 hr?

2) An eyedrop dispenser holds $\frac{1}{6}$ oz of eyedrop solution. How many dispensers can be filled from a container holding 9 oz of eyedrop solution?

3) How many $2\frac{3}{4}$ oz vials of medication can be filled from a bottle containing $41\frac{1}{4}$ oz?

4) It takes about $\frac{1}{4}$ of an hour to help a patient bathe. How many patients can an attendant help bathe in $2\frac{1}{2}$ hours?

5) A bottle of a children's pain reliever contains 100 tablets. How many $2\frac{1}{2}$ tablet doses does it contain?

6) An nurse needs $\frac{3}{4}$ hr to complete an intake interview form with each new patient. How many $\frac{3}{4}$ hr interview forms can the nurse complete in $2\frac{1}{4}$ hr?

7) How many $1\frac{1}{2}$ tablet doses are there in a bottle of 30 tablets?

8) How many $1\frac{1}{2}$ tablet doses are there in a bottle of 25 tablets?

9) A bottle holds $7\frac{3}{4}$ oz of cough syrup. How many $\frac{1}{2}$ oz doses can a nurse give from this bottle?

10) A bottle of $31\frac{1}{2}$ oz of orange juice is divided evenly among 6 residents at an assisted living facility. How many oz did each resident receive?

EXERCISES IN SOLVING MIXED APPLICATIONS

(*Answers are on pages 148–149.*)

Solve these application problems using addition, subtraction, multiplication, and/or division. Some problems may require multiple steps.

1) $6\frac{3}{8}$ mL of medication was taken from a bottle containing $16\frac{1}{2}$ mL. How much medication is left?

2) A bottle of medication contained 36 pills. If a patient took $\frac{1}{4}$ of the pills, how many are left?

3) A child was given the following amounts of medication: $\frac{3}{4}$ oz, $\frac{5}{8}$ oz, and $\frac{7}{8}$ oz. How much medication did the child receive?

4) How many $12\frac{1}{2}$ mL doses of cough syrup are there in a 175-mL bottle?

5) Each dose of cough syrup is $12\frac{1}{2}$ mL.
    If a container holds 12 doses, how many mL of cough syrup does the container hold? (This problem is different from the previous one.)

6) The weather was very bad last Friday night. Only $\frac{3}{4}$ of the nurses showed up for work. Of the 12 nurses scheduled, how many showed up?

SECTION TEST: DIVISION OF FRACTIONS

(Answers are on pages 149–151.)

What are the reciprocals of these numbers?

1) $\frac{2}{3}$ 2) 8   3) $\frac{9}{16}$

Use division to solve these problems. Turn improper fractions into mixed numbers and reduce where possible.

4) $\frac{3}{4} \div \frac{1}{2} =$ 5) $\frac{3}{8} \div \frac{3}{4} =$

6) $\frac{4}{5} \div \frac{2}{3} =$ 7) $6 \div \frac{3}{4} =$

8) $12 \div \frac{3}{16} =$ 9) $15 \div \frac{3}{5} =$

10) $\frac{2}{3} \div 6 =$ 11) $\frac{4}{5} \div 10 =$

12) $\frac{2}{5} \div 4 =$

13) $1\frac{1}{2} \div 6 =$

14) $1\frac{3}{5} \div 4 =$

15) $2\frac{2}{3} \div 8 =$

16) $2\frac{1}{3} \div \frac{7}{9} =$

17) $1\frac{3}{5} \div \frac{8}{15} =$

18) $3\frac{2}{3} \div \frac{5}{6} =$

19) $\frac{3}{8} \div 2\frac{1}{4} =$

20) $\frac{5}{6} \div 1\frac{1}{3} =$

21) $\frac{9}{16} \div 1\frac{1}{2} =$

22) $3\frac{1}{2} \div \frac{2}{5} =$

23) $3\frac{2}{3} \div 2\frac{1}{5} =$

24) $2\frac{2}{5} \div 3\frac{1}{3} =$

25) $1\frac{3}{5} \div 1\frac{3}{5} =$

26) How many $2\frac{1}{2}$ oz doses are there in a 24-oz bottle?

27) How many $4\frac{3}{4}$ oz dispensers of hand sanitizer can be filled from a 38-oz supply?

28) How many $1\frac{1}{2}$ tablet doses are there in a 50-tablet bottle?

29) 12 cups of fruit salad were divided evenly among 18 residents. How much fruit salad did each resident get? (*Hint:* Change 12 and 18 to fractions and then divide.)

ANSWERS TO EXERCISES IN RECIPROCALS OF FRACTIONS AND WHOLE NUMBERS

(Exercises are on page 115.)

1) The reciprocal of $\frac{3}{4}$ is $\frac{4}{3}$

2) The reciprocal of $\frac{2}{5}$ is $\frac{5}{2}$

3) The reciprocal of $\frac{7}{8}$ is $\frac{8}{7}$

4) The reciprocal of $\frac{4}{9}$ is $\frac{9}{4}$

5) The reciprocal of $\frac{1}{10}$ is $\frac{10}{1}$

6) The reciprocal of $\frac{5}{7}$ is $\frac{7}{5}$

7) The reciprocal of $\frac{11}{12}$ is $\frac{12}{11}$

8) The reciprocal of $\frac{9}{16}$ is $\frac{16}{9}$

9) The reciprocal of $\frac{13}{16}$ is $\frac{16}{13}$

10) The reciprocal of 3 is $\frac{1}{3}$

11) The reciprocal of 5 is $\frac{1}{5}$

12) The reciprocal of 7 is $\frac{1}{7}$

13) The reciprocal of 12 is $\frac{1}{12}$

14) The reciprocal of 100 is $\frac{1}{100}$

15) The reciprocal of 1 is $\frac{1}{1}$

ANSWERS TO EXERCISES IN REWRITING A DIVISION PROBLEM AS MULTIPLICATION BY A RECIPROCAL

(Exercises are on page 117.)

1) $\frac{1}{2} \div \frac{3}{4}$ becomes $\frac{1}{2} \times \frac{4}{3}$

2) $\frac{3}{5} \div \frac{4}{7}$ becomes $\frac{3}{5} \times \frac{7}{4}$

3) $\frac{5}{9} \div \frac{2}{7}$ becomes $\frac{5}{9} \times \frac{7}{2}$

4) $\frac{1}{3} \div \frac{2}{5}$ becomes $\frac{1}{3} \times \frac{5}{2}$

5) $\frac{7}{8} \div \frac{7}{8}$ becomes $\frac{7}{8} \times \frac{8}{7}$

6) $8 \div 4$ becomes $\frac{8}{1} \times \frac{1}{4}$

7) $5 \div 3$ becomes $\frac{5}{1} \times \frac{1}{3}$

8) $9 \div \frac{1}{3}$ becomes $\frac{9}{1} \times \frac{3}{1}$

9) $10 \div \frac{2}{5}$ becomes $\frac{10}{1} \times \frac{5}{2}$

10) $\frac{1}{2} \div 3$ becomes $\frac{1}{2} \times \frac{1}{3}$

11) $\frac{3}{8} \div 6$ becomes $\frac{3}{8} \times \frac{1}{6}$

12) $\frac{3}{4} \div 9$ becomes $\frac{3}{4} \times \frac{1}{9}$

ANSWERS TO EXERCISES IN DIVIDING A FRACTION BY A FRACTION

(Exercises are on page 120.)

1) $\frac{3}{4} \div \frac{1}{2} = \frac{3}{\overset{}{\underset{2}{4}}} \times \frac{\overset{1}{2}}{1} = \frac{3}{2} = 1\frac{1}{2}$

2) $\frac{3}{4} \div \frac{3}{4} = \frac{\overset{1}{3}}{\underset{1}{4}} \times \frac{\overset{1}{4}}{\underset{1}{3}} = \frac{1}{1} = 1$

3) $\frac{2}{5} \div \frac{1}{2} = \frac{2}{5} \times \frac{2}{1} = \frac{4}{5}$

4) $\frac{1}{8} \div \frac{1}{3} = \frac{1}{8} \times \frac{3}{1} = \frac{3}{8}$

5) $\frac{1}{5} \div \frac{3}{5} = \frac{1}{\underset{1}{5}} \times \frac{\overset{1}{5}}{3} = \frac{1}{3}$

6) $\frac{7}{8} \div \frac{1}{8} = \frac{7}{\underset{1}{8}} \times \frac{\overset{1}{8}}{1} = \frac{7}{1} = 7$

7) $\frac{3}{5} \div \frac{2}{5} = \frac{3}{\underset{1}{5}} \times \frac{\overset{1}{5}}{2} = \frac{3}{2} = 1\frac{1}{2}$

8) $\frac{1}{2} \div \frac{5}{8} = \frac{1}{\underset{1}{2}} \times \frac{\overset{4}{8}}{5} = \frac{4}{5}$

9) $\frac{3}{8} \div \frac{1}{4} = \frac{3}{\underset{2}{8}} \times \frac{\overset{1}{4}}{1} = \frac{3}{2} = 1\frac{1}{2}$

10) $\frac{1}{3} \div \frac{2}{3} = \frac{1}{\underset{1}{3}} \times \frac{\overset{1}{3}}{2} = \frac{1}{2}$

11) $\frac{1}{4} \div \frac{4}{5} = \frac{1}{4} \times \frac{5}{4} = \frac{5}{16}$

12) $\frac{3}{4} \div \frac{2}{3} = \frac{3}{4} \times \frac{3}{2} = \frac{9}{8} = 1\frac{1}{8}$

ANSWERS TO EXERCISES IN DIVIDING A WHOLE NUMBER BY A FRACTION

(Exercises are on page 122.)

1) $4 \div \frac{1}{2} = \frac{4}{1} \times \frac{2}{1} = \frac{8}{1} = 8$

2) $3 \div \frac{1}{3} = \frac{3}{1} \times \frac{3}{1} = \frac{9}{1} = 9$

3) $6 \div \frac{2}{3} = \frac{\overset{3}{6}}{1} \times \frac{3}{\underset{1}{2}} = \frac{9}{1} = 9$

4) $10 \div \frac{5}{8} = \frac{\overset{2}{10}}{1} \times \frac{8}{\underset{1}{5}} = \frac{16}{1} = 16$

5) $12 \div \frac{3}{4} = \frac{\overset{4}{12}}{1} \times \frac{4}{\underset{1}{3}} = \frac{16}{1} = 16$

6) $12 \div \frac{3}{8} = \frac{\overset{4}{12}}{1} \times \frac{8}{\underset{1}{3}} = \frac{32}{1} = 32$

7) $5 \div \frac{1}{2} = \frac{5}{1} \times \frac{2}{1} = \frac{10}{1} = 10$

8) $14 \div \frac{7}{8} = \frac{\overset{2}{14}}{1} \times \frac{8}{\underset{1}{7}} = \frac{16}{1} = 16$

9) $2 \div \frac{2}{3} = \frac{\overset{1}{2}}{1} \times \frac{3}{\underset{1}{2}} = \frac{3}{1} = 3$

10) $1 \div \frac{5}{8} = \frac{1}{1} \times \frac{8}{5} = \frac{8}{5} = 1\frac{3}{5}$

11) $4 \div \frac{3}{8} = \frac{4}{1} \times \frac{8}{3} = \frac{32}{3} = 10\frac{2}{3}$

12) $6 \div \frac{3}{4} = \frac{\overset{2}{\cancel{6}}}{1} \times \frac{4}{\underset{1}{\cancel{3}}} = \frac{8}{1} = 8$

ANSWERS TO EXERCISES IN DIVIDING A FRACTION BY A WHOLE NUMBER

(Exercises are on page 124.)

1) $\frac{1}{4} \div 2 = \frac{1}{4} \times \frac{1}{2} = \frac{1}{8}$

2) $\frac{3}{5} \div 6 = \frac{\overset{1}{\cancel{3}}}{5} \times \frac{1}{\underset{2}{\cancel{6}}} = \frac{1}{10}$

3) $\frac{7}{8} \div 7 = \frac{\overset{1}{\cancel{7}}}{8} \times \frac{1}{\underset{1}{\cancel{7}}} = \frac{1}{8}$

4) $\frac{3}{4} \div 12 = \frac{\overset{1}{\cancel{3}}}{4} \times \frac{1}{\underset{4}{\cancel{12}}} = \frac{1}{16}$

5) $\frac{2}{3} \div 12 = \frac{\overset{1}{\cancel{2}}}{3} \times \frac{1}{\underset{6}{\cancel{12}}} = \frac{1}{18}$

6) $\frac{3}{8} \div 12 = \frac{\overset{1}{\cancel{3}}}{8} \times \frac{1}{\underset{4}{\cancel{12}}} = \frac{1}{32}$

7) $\frac{3}{4} \div 2 = \frac{3}{4} \times \frac{1}{2} = \frac{3}{8}$

8) $\frac{1}{4} \div 4 = \frac{1}{4} \times \frac{1}{4} = \frac{1}{16}$

9) $\frac{5}{8} \div 2 = \frac{5}{8} \times \frac{1}{2} = \frac{5}{16}$

10) $\frac{3}{5} \div 3 = \frac{\overset{1}{\cancel{3}}}{5} \times \frac{1}{\underset{1}{\cancel{3}}} = \frac{1}{5}$

11) $\frac{7}{8} \div 14 = \frac{7}{8} \times \frac{1}{\underset{2}{\cancel{14}}} = \frac{1}{16}$

12) $\frac{2}{3} \div 8 = \frac{2}{3} \times \frac{1}{\underset{4}{\cancel{8}}} = \frac{1}{12}$

ANSWERS TO EXERCISES IN DIVIDING A MIXED NUMBER BY A WHOLE NUMBER

(Exercises are on page 126.)

1) $1\frac{1}{2} \div 2 = \frac{3}{2} \times \frac{1}{2} = \frac{3}{4}$

2) $2\frac{2}{3} \div 4 = \frac{\overset{2}{\cancel{8}}}{3} \times \frac{1}{\underset{1}{\cancel{4}}} = \frac{2}{3}$

3) $1\frac{3}{5} \div 8 = \frac{\overset{1}{\cancel{8}}}{5} \times \frac{1}{\underset{1}{\cancel{8}}} = \frac{1}{5}$

4) $1\frac{1}{3} \div 8 = \frac{\overset{1}{\cancel{4}}}{3} \times \frac{1}{\underset{2}{\cancel{8}}} = \frac{1}{6}$

5) $1\frac{7}{8} \div 5 = \frac{\overset{3}{\cancel{15}}}{8} \times \frac{1}{\underset{1}{\cancel{5}}} = \frac{3}{8}$

6) $1\frac{1}{2} \div 5 = \frac{3}{2} \times \frac{1}{5} = \frac{3}{10}$

7) $2\frac{2}{3} \div 8 = \frac{\overset{1}{\cancel{8}}}{3} \times \frac{1}{\underset{1}{\cancel{8}}} = \frac{1}{3}$

8) $1\frac{3}{5} \div 4 = \frac{\overset{2}{\cancel{8}}}{5} \times \frac{1}{\underset{1}{\cancel{4}}} = \frac{2}{5}$

9) $5\frac{2}{5} \div 9 = \frac{\overset{3}{\cancel{27}}}{5} \times \frac{1}{\underset{1}{\cancel{9}}} = \frac{3}{5}$

10) $1\frac{1}{2} \div 9 = \frac{\overset{1}{\cancel{3}}}{2} \times \frac{1}{\underset{3}{\cancel{9}}} = \frac{1}{6}$

11) $2\frac{3}{4} \div 11 = \frac{\overset{1}{\cancel{11}}}{4} \times \frac{1}{\underset{1}{\cancel{11}}} = \frac{1}{4}$

12) $2\frac{2}{3} \div 12 = \frac{\overset{2}{\cancel{8}}}{3} \times \frac{1}{\underset{3}{\cancel{12}}} = \frac{2}{9}$

ANSWERS TO EXERCISES IN DIVIDING A MIXED NUMBER BY A FRACTION

(Exercises are on page 128.)

1) $1\frac{1}{2} \div \frac{1}{3} = \frac{3}{2} \times \frac{3}{1} = \frac{9}{2} = 4\frac{1}{2}$

2) $1\frac{3}{4} \div \frac{1}{2} = \frac{7}{\underset{2}{\cancel{4}}} \times \frac{\overset{1}{\cancel{2}}}{1} = \frac{7}{2} = 3\frac{1}{2}$

3) $1\frac{1}{2} \div \frac{3}{4} = \frac{\overset{1}{\cancel{3}}}{\underset{1}{\cancel{2}}} \times \frac{\overset{2}{\cancel{4}}}{\underset{1}{\cancel{3}}} = \frac{2}{1} = 2$

4) $1\frac{1}{4} \div \frac{3}{8} = \frac{5}{\underset{1}{\cancel{4}}} \times \frac{\overset{2}{\cancel{8}}}{3} = \frac{10}{3} = 3\frac{1}{3}$

5) $1\frac{1}{2} \div \frac{3}{8} = \frac{\overset{1}{\cancel{3}}}{\underset{1}{\cancel{2}}} \times \frac{\overset{4}{\cancel{8}}}{\underset{1}{\cancel{3}}} = \frac{4}{1} = 4$

6) $2\frac{3}{4} \div \frac{2}{5} = \frac{11}{4} \times \frac{5}{2} = \frac{55}{8} = 6\frac{7}{8}$

7) $2\frac{3}{4} \div \frac{1}{2} = \frac{11}{\underset{2}{\cancel{4}}} \times \frac{\overset{1}{\cancel{2}}}{1} = \frac{11}{2} = 5\frac{1}{2}$

8) $2\frac{2}{3} \div \frac{4}{5} = \frac{\overset{2}{\cancel{8}}}{3} \times \frac{5}{\underset{1}{\cancel{4}}} = \frac{10}{3} = 3\frac{1}{3}$

9) $2\frac{5}{8} \div \frac{7}{8} = \frac{\overset{3}{\cancel{21}}}{\underset{1}{\cancel{8}}} \times \frac{\overset{1}{\cancel{8}}}{\underset{1}{\cancel{7}}} = \frac{3}{1} = 3$

10) $3\frac{1}{2} \div 1\frac{2}{5} = \frac{7}{2} \times \frac{5}{\underset{1}{\cancel{7}}} = \frac{5}{2} = 2\frac{1}{2}$

11) $3\frac{2}{3} \div 2\frac{1}{5} = \frac{\overset{1}{\cancel{11}}}{3} \times \frac{5}{\underset{1}{\cancel{11}}} = \frac{5}{3} = 1\frac{2}{3}$

12) $2\frac{2}{5} \div 3\frac{1}{3} = \frac{\overset{6}{\cancel{12}}}{5} \times \frac{3}{\underset{5}{\cancel{10}}} = \frac{18}{25}$

ANSWERS TO EXERCISES IN DIVIDING A FRACTION BY A MIXED NUMBER

(Exercises are on page 130.)

1) $\dfrac{1}{2} \div 1\dfrac{1}{2} = \dfrac{1}{\overset{}{\underset{1}{2}}} \times \dfrac{\overset{1}{2}}{3} = \dfrac{1}{3}$

2) $\dfrac{4}{5} \div 1\dfrac{1}{3} = \dfrac{\overset{1}{4}}{5} \times \dfrac{3}{\underset{1}{4}} = \dfrac{3}{5}$

3) $\dfrac{3}{4} \div 1\dfrac{1}{2} = \dfrac{\overset{1}{3}}{\underset{2}{4}} \times \dfrac{\overset{1}{2}}{3} = \dfrac{1}{2}$

4) $\dfrac{7}{8} \div 2\dfrac{5}{8} = \dfrac{7}{\underset{1}{8}} \times \dfrac{\overset{1}{8}}{\underset{3}{21}} = \dfrac{1}{3}$

5) $\dfrac{3}{4} \div 1\dfrac{1}{4} = \dfrac{3}{\underset{1}{4}} \times \dfrac{\overset{1}{4}}{5} = \dfrac{3}{5}$

6) $\dfrac{5}{8} \div 1\dfrac{2}{3} = \dfrac{\overset{1}{5}}{8} \times \dfrac{3}{\underset{1}{5}} = \dfrac{3}{8}$

7) $\dfrac{3}{5} \div 1\dfrac{1}{2} = \dfrac{\overset{1}{3}}{5} \times \dfrac{2}{\underset{1}{3}} = \dfrac{2}{5}$

8) $\dfrac{4}{5} \div 2\dfrac{2}{3} = \dfrac{\overset{1}{4}}{5} \times \dfrac{3}{\underset{2}{8}} = \dfrac{3}{10}$

9) $\dfrac{5}{8} \div 1\dfrac{1}{4} = \dfrac{\overset{1}{5}}{\underset{1}{8}} \times \dfrac{\overset{1}{4}}{\underset{1}{5}} = \dfrac{1}{2}$

10) $\dfrac{2}{3} \div 1\dfrac{2}{3} = \dfrac{2}{\underset{1}{3}} \times \dfrac{\overset{1}{3}}{5} = \dfrac{2}{5}$

11) $\dfrac{3}{4} \div 1\dfrac{7}{8} = \dfrac{\overset{1}{3}}{\underset{1}{4}} \times \dfrac{\overset{2}{8}}{\underset{5}{15}} = \dfrac{2}{5}$

12) $\dfrac{2}{5} \div 3\dfrac{3}{5} = \dfrac{\overset{1}{2}}{\underset{1}{5}} \times \dfrac{\overset{1}{5}}{\underset{9}{18}} = \dfrac{1}{9}$

ANSWERS TO EXERCISES IN DIVIDING A MIXED NUMBER BY A MIXED NUMBER

(Exercises are on page 132.)

1) $1\dfrac{1}{8} \div 2\dfrac{1}{4} = \dfrac{9}{8} \div \dfrac{9}{4} = \dfrac{\overset{1}{9}}{\underset{2}{8}} \times \dfrac{\overset{1}{4}}{\underset{1}{9}} = \dfrac{1}{2}$

2) $1\dfrac{4}{5} \div 4\dfrac{1}{2} = \dfrac{9}{5} \div \dfrac{9}{2} = \dfrac{\overset{1}{9}}{5} \times \dfrac{2}{\underset{1}{9}} = \dfrac{2}{5}$

3) $1\dfrac{1}{4} \div 1\dfrac{7}{8} = \dfrac{5}{4} \div \dfrac{15}{8} = \dfrac{\overset{1}{5}}{\underset{1}{4}} \times \dfrac{\overset{2}{8}}{\underset{3}{15}} = \dfrac{2}{3}$

4) $2\dfrac{3}{4} \div 3\dfrac{3}{4} = \dfrac{11}{4} \div \dfrac{15}{4} = \dfrac{11}{\underset{1}{4}} \times \dfrac{\overset{1}{4}}{15} = \dfrac{11}{15}$

5) $4\frac{2}{3} \div 2\frac{1}{3} = \frac{14}{3} \div \frac{7}{3} = \frac{\overset{2}{\cancel{14}}}{\underset{1}{\cancel{3}}} \times \frac{\overset{1}{\cancel{3}}}{\cancel{7}} = \frac{2}{1} = 2$

6) $1\frac{3}{7} \div 1\frac{2}{3} = \frac{10}{7} \div \frac{5}{3} = \frac{\overset{2}{\cancel{10}}}{7} \times \frac{3}{\underset{1}{\cancel{5}}} = \frac{6}{7}$

7) $2\frac{2}{3} \div 1\frac{7}{9} = \frac{8}{3} \div \frac{16}{9} = \frac{\overset{1}{\cancel{8}}}{\underset{1}{\cancel{3}}} \times \frac{\overset{3}{\cancel{9}}}{\underset{2}{\cancel{16}}} = \frac{3}{2} = 1\frac{1}{2}$

8) $5\frac{5}{8} \div 1\frac{1}{4} = \frac{45}{8} \div \frac{5}{4} = \frac{\overset{9}{\cancel{45}}}{\underset{2}{\cancel{8}}} \times \frac{\overset{1}{\cancel{4}}}{\cancel{5}} = \frac{9}{2} = 4\frac{1}{2}$

9) $1\frac{1}{4} \div 3\frac{1}{8} = \frac{5}{4} \div \frac{25}{8} = \frac{\overset{1}{\cancel{5}}}{\underset{1}{\cancel{4}}} \times \frac{\overset{2}{\cancel{8}}}{\underset{5}{\cancel{25}}} = \frac{2}{5}$

10) $2\frac{2}{5} \div 1\frac{1}{5} = \frac{12}{5} \div \frac{6}{5} = \frac{\overset{2}{\cancel{12}}}{\underset{1}{\cancel{5}}} \times \frac{\overset{1}{\cancel{5}}}{\underset{1}{\cancel{6}}} = \frac{2}{1} = 2$

11) $2\frac{2}{3} \div 4\frac{4}{5} = \frac{8}{3} \div \frac{24}{5} = \frac{\overset{1}{\cancel{8}}}{3} \times \frac{5}{\underset{3}{\cancel{24}}} = \frac{5}{9}$

12) $4\frac{2}{3} \div 1\frac{2}{5} = \frac{14}{3} \div \frac{7}{5} = \frac{\overset{2}{\cancel{14}}}{3} \times \frac{5}{\underset{1}{\cancel{7}}} = \frac{10}{3} = 3\frac{1}{3}$

ANSWERS TO EXERCISES IN SOLVING DIVISION APPLICATIONS

(*Exercises are on pages 134–135.*)

1)   The 3 hr is being divided into units of $\frac{1}{3}$ hr each. $3 \div \frac{1}{3} = \frac{3}{1} \times \frac{3}{1} = 9$
Thus, 9 patients can be groomed in 3 hours.

2)   The 9 oz of eyedrop solution in the container has to be divided into $\frac{1}{6}$ oz units.
$9 \div \frac{1}{6} = \frac{9}{1} \times \frac{6}{1} = \frac{54}{1} = 54$. The 9 oz in the container will fill 54 dispensers.

3) Divide the $41\frac{1}{4}$ oz in the container by the $2\frac{3}{4}$ oz in each vial to find how many vials the container will fill.

$$41\frac{1}{4} \div 2\frac{3}{4} = \frac{165}{4} \div \frac{11}{4} = \frac{165}{\overset{1}{\cancel{4}}} \times \frac{\overset{1}{\cancel{4}}}{11} = \frac{165}{11} = 15$$

The container will fill 15 $2\frac{3}{4}$ oz vials.

4) Divide the $2\frac{1}{2}$ hr by the $\frac{1}{4}$ hr it takes to bathe one patient to calculate how many patients can be bathed in this amount of time.

$$2\frac{1}{2} \div \frac{1}{4} = \frac{5}{\underset{1}{\cancel{2}}} \times \frac{\overset{2}{\cancel{4}}}{1} = \frac{5 \times 2}{1 \times 1} = \frac{10}{1} = 10.$$ The attendant can bathe 10 patients.

5) Divide the 100 tablets of pain reliever by the $2\frac{1}{2}$ tablets needed for each dose to find how many doses the bottle contains.

$$100 \div 2\frac{1}{2} = \frac{\overset{20}{\cancel{100}}}{1} \times \frac{2}{\underset{1}{\cancel{5}}} = \frac{20 \times 2}{1 \times 1} = \frac{40}{1} = 40.$$ The bottle contains 40 of the $2\frac{1}{2}$ tablet doses.

6) Divide the total amount of time ($2\frac{1}{4}$ hr) the nurse has by the $\frac{3}{4}$ hr he needs to complete each interview form to get how many forms he can do.

$$2\frac{1}{4} \div \frac{3}{4} = \frac{\overset{3}{\cancel{9}}}{\underset{1}{\cancel{4}}} \times \frac{\overset{1}{\cancel{4}}}{\underset{1}{\cancel{3}}} = \frac{3}{1} = 3.$$ The nurse can complete 3 interview forms.

7) Divide the number of tablets (30) by the amount of one dose $\left(1\frac{1}{2}\right)$ to find the total number of doses in the bottle.

$$30 \div 1\frac{1}{2} = \frac{\overset{10}{\cancel{30}}}{1} \times \frac{2}{\underset{1}{\cancel{3}}} = \frac{10 \times 2}{1 \times 1} = \frac{20}{1} = 20.$$ There are 20 of the $1\frac{1}{2}$ tablet doses in the bottle.

8) Solve this problem just like the previous problem. Divide the number of tablets (25) by the amount of one dose $\left(1\frac{1}{2}\right)$ to find the total number of doses in the bottle.

$$25 \div 1\frac{1}{2} = \frac{25}{1} \times \frac{2}{3} = \frac{25 \times 2}{1 \times 3} = \frac{50}{3} = 16\frac{2}{3}.$$ A partial dose would not be given, so there are 16 of the $1\frac{1}{2}$ tablet doses in the bottle.

9) Divide the $7\frac{3}{4}$ oz of cough syrup in the bottle by $\frac{1}{2}$ oz for each dose to get the total number of doses in the bottle.

$$7\frac{3}{4} \div \frac{1}{2} = \frac{31}{\overset{}{\cancel{4}}} \times \frac{\overset{1}{\cancel{2}}}{1} = \frac{31 \times 1}{2 \times 1} = \frac{31}{2} = 15\frac{1}{2}.$$ A partial dose would not be given, so there are 15 of the $\frac{1}{2}$ oz doses in the bottle.

10) Divide the $31\frac{1}{2}$ oz of orange juice by the 6 residents to find how many oz each resident received.

$$31\frac{1}{2} \div 6 = \frac{\overset{21}{\cancel{63}}}{2} \div \frac{1}{\underset{2}{\cancel{6}}} = \frac{21 \times 1}{2 \times 2} = \frac{21}{4} = 5\frac{1}{4}.$$ Each resident received $5\frac{1}{4}$ oz of orange juice.

ANSWERS TO EXERCISES IN SOLVING MIXED APPLICATIONS

(*Exercises are on pages 136–137.*)

1)
$$16\frac{1}{2} = 16\frac{4}{8}$$
$$\underline{-6\frac{3}{8} = 6\frac{3}{8}}$$
$$10\frac{1}{8}$$

Subtract the amount of medication taken from the bottle from the original amount to find how much medication is left. There are $10\frac{1}{8}$ mL of medication left in the bottle.

2) First, multiply the number of pills (36) times $\frac{1}{4}$ to find how many pills the patient took. Then, subtract the number of pills the patient took from the original amount to find how many pills are left. The patient took 9 pills, so there are 27 pills left in the bottle.

First: $36 \times \frac{1}{4} = \frac{\overset{9}{\cancel{36}}}{1} \times \frac{1}{\underset{1}{\cancel{4}}} = \frac{1 \times 9}{1 \times 1} = \frac{9}{1} = 9$ Then $36 - 9 = 27$.

3)
$$\frac{3}{4} = \frac{6}{8}$$
$$\frac{5}{8} = \frac{5}{8}$$
$$\underline{+\frac{7}{8} = \frac{7}{8}}$$
$$\frac{18}{8} = 2\frac{2}{8} = 2\frac{1}{4}$$

Add the amounts of medication to get the total amount of medication the child received. The child received $2\frac{1}{4}$ oz of medication.

4) Divide the 175 mL of cough syrup in the bottle by the dose of $12\frac{1}{2}$ mL to find how many doses the bottle contains. The bottle contains 14 of the $12\frac{1}{2}$ mL doses.

$$175 \div 12\frac{1}{2} = \frac{175}{1} \div \frac{25}{2} = \frac{175}{1} \times \frac{2}{25} = \frac{\overset{7}{\cancel{175}}}{1} \times \frac{2}{\underset{1}{\cancel{25}}} = \frac{7 \times 2}{1 \times 1} = \frac{14}{1} = 14$$

5) Multiply the amount of each dose times the number of doses in the container to find how many mL the container holds. The container holds 150 mL.

$$12\frac{1}{2} \times 12 = \frac{25}{2} \times \frac{12}{1} = \frac{25}{\underset{1}{\cancel{2}}} \times \frac{\overset{6}{\cancel{12}}}{1} = \frac{25 \times 6}{1 \times 1} = \frac{150}{1} = 150$$

6) Multiply the fraction of nurses that showed times the number of nurses that were scheduled to find how many of the nurses showed for work. 9 nurses showed for work.

$$\frac{3}{4} \times 12 = \frac{3}{\cancel{4}_1} \times \frac{\cancel{12}^3}{1} = \frac{3 \times 3}{1 \times 1} = \frac{9}{1} = 9$$

ANSWERS TO SECTION TEST: DIVISION OF FRACTIONS

(*Section Test is on pages 138–140.*)

1) The reciprocal of $\frac{2}{3}$ is $\frac{3}{2}$

2) The reciprocal of 8 is $\frac{1}{8}$

3) The reciprocal of $\frac{9}{16}$ is $\frac{16}{9}$

4) $\frac{3}{4} \div \frac{1}{2} = \frac{3}{\cancel{4}_2} \times \frac{\cancel{2}^1}{1} = \frac{3 \times 1}{2 \times 1} = \frac{3}{2} = 1\frac{1}{2}$

5) $\frac{3}{8} \div \frac{3}{4} = \frac{\cancel{3}^1}{\cancel{8}_2} \times \frac{\cancel{4}^1}{\cancel{3}_1} = \frac{1 \times 1}{2 \times 1} = \frac{1}{2}$

6) $\frac{4}{5} \div \frac{2}{3} = \frac{\cancel{4}^2}{5} \times \frac{3}{\cancel{2}_1} = \frac{2 \times 3}{5 \times 1} = \frac{6}{5} = 1\frac{1}{5}$

7) $6 \div \frac{3}{4} = \frac{6}{1} \div \frac{3}{4} = \frac{\cancel{6}^2}{1} \times \frac{4}{\cancel{3}_1} = \frac{2 \times 4}{1 \times 1} = \frac{8}{1} = 8$

8) $12 \div \frac{3}{16} = \frac{12}{1} \div \frac{3}{16} = \frac{\cancel{12}^4}{1} \times \frac{16}{\cancel{3}_1} = \frac{4 \times 16}{1 \times 1} = \frac{64}{1} = 64$

9) $15 \div \frac{3}{5} = \frac{15}{1} \div \frac{3}{5} = \frac{\cancel{15}^5}{1} \times \frac{5}{\cancel{3}_1} = \frac{5 \times 5}{1 \times 1} = \frac{25}{1} = 25$

10) $\frac{2}{3} \div 6 = \frac{2}{3} \div \frac{6}{1} = \frac{\cancel{2}^1}{3} \times \frac{1}{\cancel{6}_3} = \frac{1 \times 1}{3 \times 3} = \frac{1}{9}$

11) $\dfrac{4}{5} \div 10 = \dfrac{4}{5} \div \dfrac{10}{1} = \dfrac{\overset{2}{\cancel{4}}}{5} \times \dfrac{1}{\underset{5}{\cancel{10}}} = \dfrac{2 \times 1}{5 \times 5} = \dfrac{2}{25}$

12) $\dfrac{2}{5} \div 4 = \dfrac{2}{5} \div \dfrac{4}{1} = \dfrac{\overset{1}{\cancel{2}}}{5} \times \dfrac{1}{\underset{2}{\cancel{4}}} = \dfrac{1 \times 1}{5 \times 2} = \dfrac{1}{10}$

13) $1\dfrac{1}{2} \div 6 = \dfrac{3}{2} \div \dfrac{6}{1} = \dfrac{\overset{1}{\cancel{3}}}{2} \times \dfrac{1}{\underset{2}{\cancel{6}}} = \dfrac{1 \times 1}{2 \times 2} = \dfrac{1}{4}$

14) $1\dfrac{3}{5} \div 4 = \dfrac{8}{5} \div \dfrac{4}{1} = \dfrac{\overset{2}{\cancel{8}}}{5} \times \dfrac{1}{\underset{1}{\cancel{4}}} = \dfrac{2 \times 1}{5 \times 1} = \dfrac{2}{5}$

15) $2\dfrac{2}{3} \div 8 = \dfrac{8}{3} \div \dfrac{8}{1} = \dfrac{\overset{1}{\cancel{8}}}{3} \times \dfrac{1}{\underset{1}{\cancel{8}}} = \dfrac{1 \times 1}{3 \times 1} = \dfrac{1}{3}$

16) $2\dfrac{1}{3} \div \dfrac{7}{9} = \dfrac{7}{3} \div \dfrac{7}{9} = \dfrac{\overset{1}{\cancel{7}}}{\underset{1}{\cancel{3}}} \times \dfrac{\overset{3}{\cancel{9}}}{\cancel{7}} = \dfrac{1 \times 3}{1 \times 1} = \dfrac{3}{1} = 3$

17) $1\dfrac{3}{5} \div \dfrac{8}{15} = \dfrac{8}{5} \div \dfrac{8}{15} = \dfrac{\overset{1}{\cancel{8}}}{\underset{1}{\cancel{5}}} \times \dfrac{\overset{3}{\cancel{15}}}{\underset{1}{\cancel{8}}} = \dfrac{1 \times 3}{1 \times 1} = \dfrac{3}{1} = 3$

18) $3\dfrac{2}{3} \div \dfrac{5}{6} = \dfrac{11}{3} \div \dfrac{5}{6} = \dfrac{11}{\underset{1}{\cancel{3}}} \times \dfrac{\overset{2}{\cancel{6}}}{5} = \dfrac{11 \times 2}{1 \times 5} = \dfrac{22}{5} = 4\dfrac{2}{5}$

19) $\dfrac{3}{8} \div 2\dfrac{1}{4} = \dfrac{3}{8} \div \dfrac{9}{4} = \dfrac{\overset{1}{\cancel{3}}}{\underset{2}{\cancel{8}}} \times \dfrac{\overset{1}{\cancel{4}}}{\underset{3}{\cancel{9}}} = \dfrac{1 \times 1}{2 \times 3} = \dfrac{1}{6}$

20) $\dfrac{5}{6} \div 1\dfrac{1}{3} = \dfrac{5}{6} \div \dfrac{4}{3} = \dfrac{5}{\underset{2}{\cancel{6}}} \times \dfrac{\overset{1}{\cancel{3}}}{4} = \dfrac{5 \times 1}{2 \times 4} = \dfrac{5}{8}$

21) $\dfrac{9}{16} \div 1\dfrac{1}{2} = \dfrac{9}{16} \div \dfrac{3}{2} = \dfrac{\overset{3}{\cancel{9}}}{\underset{8}{\cancel{16}}} \times \dfrac{\overset{1}{\cancel{2}}}{\underset{1}{\cancel{3}}} = \dfrac{3 \times 1}{8 \times 1} = \dfrac{3}{8}$

22) $3\dfrac{1}{2} \div \dfrac{2}{5} = \dfrac{7}{2} \div \dfrac{2}{5} = \dfrac{7}{2} \times \dfrac{5}{2} = \dfrac{7 \times 5}{2 \times 2} = \dfrac{35}{4} = 8\dfrac{3}{4}$

23) $3\frac{2}{3} \div 2\frac{1}{5} = \frac{11}{3} \div \frac{11}{5} = \frac{\overset{1}{\cancel{11}}}{3} \times \frac{5}{\cancel{11}} = \frac{1 \times 5}{3 \times 1} = \frac{5}{3} = 1\frac{2}{3}$

24) $2\frac{2}{5} \div 3\frac{1}{3} = \frac{12}{5} \div \frac{10}{3} = \frac{\overset{6}{\cancel{12}}}{5} \times \frac{3}{\underset{5}{\cancel{10}}} = \frac{6 \times 3}{5 \times 5} = \frac{18}{25}$

25) $1\frac{3}{5} \div 1\frac{3}{5} = \frac{8}{5} \div \frac{8}{5} = \frac{\overset{1}{\cancel{8}}}{\underset{1}{\cancel{5}}} \times \frac{\overset{1}{\cancel{5}}}{\underset{1}{\cancel{8}}} = \frac{1 \times 1}{1 \times 1} = \frac{1}{1} = 1$

Any number divided by itself is 1.

26) Divide the 24 oz in the bottle by the $2\frac{1}{2}$ oz of each dose to find out how many doses there are in the bottle.

$24 \div 2\frac{1}{2} = \frac{24}{1} \div \frac{5}{2} = \frac{24}{1} \times \frac{2}{5} = \frac{24 \times 2}{1 \times 5} = \frac{48}{5} = 9\frac{3}{5}$

There are 9 of the $2\frac{1}{2}$ oz doses in the bottle. The partial dose would not be given.

27) Divide the 38-oz supply of hand sanitizer by the $4\frac{3}{4}$ oz for each dispenser to calculate how many dispensers can be filled.

$38 \div 4\frac{3}{4} = \frac{38}{1} \div \frac{19}{4} = \frac{\overset{2}{\cancel{38}}}{1} \times \frac{4}{\underset{1}{\cancel{19}}} = \frac{2 \times 4}{1 \times 1} = \frac{8}{1} = 8$

A total of 8 of the $4\frac{3}{4}$ oz dispensers can be filled from this supply.

28) Divide the 50 tablets in the bottle by the $1\frac{1}{2}$ tablets in each dose to calculate how many doses are in the bottle.

$50 \div 1\frac{1}{2} = \frac{50}{1} \div \frac{3}{2} = \frac{50}{1} \times \frac{2}{3} = \frac{50 \times 2}{1 \times 3} = \frac{100}{3} = 33\frac{1}{3}$

There are 33 of the $1\frac{1}{2}$ tablet doses in the bottle. The partial dose would not be given.

29) Divide the 12 cups of fruit salad by the 18 residents to calculate how much each resident would receive.

$12 \div 18 = \frac{12}{1} \div \frac{18}{1} = \frac{\overset{2}{\cancel{12}}}{1} \times \frac{1}{\underset{3}{\cancel{18}}} = \frac{2 \times 1}{1 \times 3} = \frac{2}{3}$

Each resident would receive $\frac{2}{3}$ cup of fruit salad.

What Is a Fraction?

A **fraction** is a method of division and is used to indicate a part of a whole. A fraction consists of an upper number called the **numerator** and a lower number called the **denominator**. They are separated by a horizontal line. For the fraction $\frac{3}{4}$, the denominator 4 indicates that 1 whole unit is divided into 4 parts. The numerator 3 indicates that this fraction consists of three of the 4 parts.

To reduce a fraction to its lowest terms

If a number can divide evenly into both the numerator and the denominator of a fraction without having a remainder, then the fraction can be reduced by that number.

If there is no number that can divide evenly into both the numerator and the denominator, then the fraction cannot be reduced. If a fraction cannot be reduced, the fraction is in its **lowest terms**. A final answer should have a fraction reduced to its lowest terms.

The three forms of fractions

There are three forms or types of fractions: proper fractions, improper fractions, and mixed numbers. A **proper fraction** has a denominator that is larger than the numerator. $\frac{3}{5}$ is an example of a proper fraction. An **improper fraction** has a numerator that is equal to or larger than the denominator. $\frac{5}{3}$ and $\frac{4}{4}$ are examples of improper fractions. When the numerator and denominator are equal, the fraction can be reduced to 1. A **mixed number** is a combination of a whole number and a fraction. $1\frac{2}{3}$ is an example of a mixed number.

To change an improper fraction to a whole number or a mixed number

Step 1: Divide the denominator into the numerator. The answer (without the remainder) is the whole-number part of the mixed number.

Step 2: Write the remainder part of the answer as the numerator with the divisor of the fraction as the denominator. If there is no remainder, the answer is just a whole number.

Step 3: Reduce the fraction if possible.

Note: If there is no remainder, the answer is a whole number, not a mixed number.

To turn $\frac{5}{3}$ into a mixed number, divide 3 into 5.

$$\begin{array}{r} 1 \\ 3\overline{)5} \\ \underline{3} \\ 2 \end{array}$$ 3 goes into 5 one time with a remainder of 2. The whole number in the mixed number is 1, the numerator of the fraction is 2, and the denominator of the fraction is 3.

Thus, $\frac{5}{3}$ as a mixed number is $1\frac{2}{3}$.

To change a whole number to an improper fraction

To change a whole number to an improper fraction, place the whole number in the numerator and use a denominator of 1. To change 6 to an improper fraction, place 6 in the numerator and use a denominator of 1. Thus, $6 = \frac{6}{1}$.

To change a mixed number to an improper fraction

Step 1: Multiply the denominator times the whole-number part of the mixed number.

Step 2: Add the answer from Step 1 to the numerator of the mixed number.

Step 3: Place this total over the same denominator of the mixed number.

To change $2\frac{3}{4}$ to an improper fraction, multiply the denominator, which is 4, times the whole number 2 to get 8. Next, add 8 to the numerator 3 to get a total of 11. Place 11 in the numerator with the original denominator of 4. Thus, $2\frac{3}{4} = \frac{11}{4}$.

To add fractions with like denominators

To add fractions with like denominators, add the numerators and use the same denominator. For example, 2 and 3 equal 5: $\frac{2}{7} + \frac{3}{7} = \frac{5}{7}$. Frequently, when adding fractions, the answer may have to be changed to a mixed number and reduced.

To find the least common multiple of a set of numbers

The **common multiples** of a set of numbers are multiples that can be divided evenly by all of the numbers in the set.

Consider the set of 3 and 2. Their multiples are:

Multiples of 3: 3, <u>6</u>, 9, <u>12</u>, 15, <u>18</u>, 21 ...

Multiples of 2: 2, 4, <u>6</u>, 8, 10, <u>12</u>, 14, 16, <u>18</u>, 20 ...

The numbers they share in common from this list are 6, 12, and 18. The lowest number is 6. This is called the *least common multiple*.

The **least common multiple** of a set of numbers is the lowest multiple into which all of the numbers in the set can divide evenly. Use the least common multiple as the lowest common denominator for a group of fractions. The **lowest common denominator** (**LCD**) is the smallest number that can be divided evenly by all of the denominators in the group of fractions.

To raise a fraction to a higher term

If a number is multiplied by both the numerator and the denominator, the fraction is raised to a higher term. The amount the fraction represents does not change. This is the opposite of reducing a fraction.

To raise a fraction to a higher term, multiply the numerator and the denominator by the same number.

To add fractions with unlike denominators

Step 1: Find the lowest common denominator for the fractions to be added.

Step 2: Change one or more of the fractions so they have the same denominators.

Step 3: Add the fractions.

Step 4: If necessary, change the answer to a mixed number and reduce when possible.

To add mixed numbers with like denominators

To add mixed numbers with like denominators, add the fractions and the whole numbers separately. If the fraction part of the answer is an improper fraction, change it to a mixed number and add the whole numbers. Reduce if possible.

To add mixed numbers with unlike denominators

Step 1: Change the fractions so they have like denominators.

Step 2: Next, add the fractions and the whole numbers separately. If the fraction part of the answer is an improper fraction, change it to a mixed number and add the whole numbers. Reduce if possible.

To solve addition applications

Use addition to answer questions that ask for the total or how much something is all together. For the addition process, smaller amounts are combined into a larger amount.

The following key words may indicate the need to add: *total, sum, and, plus, all, altogether, entire, added to,* and *with tax*.

If your answer is an improper fraction, convert it to a mixed number. Reduce if possible. Include the label in the answer.

To subtract fractions with like denominators

The answer to a subtraction problem is called the **difference**. To subtract fractions with the same denominators, subtract the numerators and put the difference over the same denominator. Check the answer by using addition.

To subtract fractions with unlike denominators without borrowing

Step 1: Find the lowest common denominator for the fractions.

Step 2: Change one or more of the fractions so the fractions all have the same denominator.

Step 3: Subtract the fractions.

To subtract mixed numbers with unlike denominators without borrowing

Step 1: Find the lowest common denominator for the fractions.

Step 2: Change one or more of the fractions so they have the same denominator.

Step 3: Subtract the fractions and subtract the whole numbers.

To convert 1 to a fraction with a specific denominator

Step 1: Change 1 to a fraction of $\frac{1}{1}$.

Step 2: Raise this fraction to a fraction with the denominator needed. If the denominator is 3, then the fraction becomes $\frac{3}{3}$.

To subtract a fraction from a whole number

Step 1: Borrow 1 from the whole number and change it to a fraction, creating a mixed number.

Step 2: Change the fraction so it has the same denominator as the fraction to be subtracted.

Step 3: Subtract the fraction from the mixed number.

To borrow 1 from a mixed number

Step 1: Borrow 1 from the whole number and change it to the same denominator as the fraction in the mixed number.

Step 2: Add the two fractions together.

To subtract fractions using borrowing

Step 1: Change both fractions to the same denominator if necessary.

Step 2: Borrow 1 from the whole number and change it to the same denominator as the fraction in the mixed number. Add the two fractions together.

Step 3: Subtract the fractions and the whole numbers.

To solve subtraction applications

Use subtraction to answer questions that ask for the difference between two numbers. For the subtraction process, a smaller amount is removed from the original amount.

The following key words may indicate the need to subtract: *how much greater than; how much less than; how much of an increase or decrease; how many more; how much farther, or bigger, or smaller, or heavier,* and so on.

If your answer is an improper fraction, convert it to a mixed number. Reduce if possible. Include the label in the answer.

To multiply two fractions together

To multiply two fractions together, multiply the numerators together and multiply the denominators together. Reduce the answer if possible.

To use canceling when multiplying fractions

Canceling is a method of reducing fractions before they are multiplied. When canceling fractions that are multiplied together, reduce any one of the numerators with any one of the denominators. Continue reducing other numerators and denominators until no more reducing can be done. Multiply the fractions.

To multiply whole numbers and fractions

To multiply a whole number times a fraction, convert the whole number to a fraction by placing the number over a denominator of one. Cancel when possible, and then multiply the fractions.

To multiply mixed numbers

To multiply mixed numbers, convert the mixed numbers to improper fractions. Cancel when possible, and then multiply the fractions.

To solve multiplication applications

Multiplication application problems generally give information about one item and ask for information representing several of these items.

The following key words may indicate the need to multiply: *product, times, of,* or *multiplied by.*

For instance, if one shirt costs $5, how much would 3 shirts cost? To solve this, multiply the cost of one shirt ($5) by the number of shirts (3) to get the cost of those shirts ($15).

To create a reciprocal of a fraction

A **reciprocal** of a fraction is its inverse. The numerator in the fraction is used as the denominator of the reciprocal, and the denominator of the fraction is used as the numerator of the reciprocal. For example, the reciprocal of $\frac{2}{3}$ is $\frac{3}{2}$.

A fraction multiplied by its reciprocal equals 1: $\overset{1}{\underset{1}{\frac{2}{3}}} \times \overset{1}{\underset{1}{\frac{3}{2}}} = \frac{1}{1} = 1.$

To create a reciprocal of a whole number

To find the reciprocal of a whole number, turn the whole number into a fraction and then create its reciprocal. To find the reciprocal of 2, turn 2 into the fraction $\frac{2}{1}$. The reciprocal of $\frac{2}{1}$ is $\frac{1}{2}$.

To rewrite a division problem as multiplication of a reciprocal

Dividing by a number will give the same answer as multiplying by the number's reciprocal. Example: $6 \div 2 = 3$. Because the reciprocal of 2 is $\frac{1}{2}$, multiplying 6 times $\frac{1}{2}$ will give same answer: $6 \times \frac{1}{2} = \frac{\overset{3}{\cancel{6}}}{1} \times \frac{1}{\underset{1}{\cancel{2}}} = \frac{3}{1} = 3$. Because of this, when working with fractions, instead of dividing, we multiply by the reciprocal of the divisor.

To rewrite a division problem as multiplication by a reciprocal, do these steps.

Step 1: Leave the first number as it is.

Step 2: Change the division sign to the multiplication sign.

Step 3: Find the reciprocal of the divisor (the number after the division sign). Change the divisor to its reciprocal.

To divide a fraction by a fraction

Instead of dividing by a fraction, multiply by the reciprocal of the fraction. In other words, change the division sign to multiplication and multiply by the reciprocal of the divisor.

To divide a whole number by a fraction

To divide a whole number by a fraction, turn the whole number into its equivalent fraction. Next, multiply by the reciprocal of the divisor.

To divide a fraction by a whole number

To divide a fraction by a whole number, turn the whole number into its equivalent fraction. Next, multiply by the reciprocal of that fraction.

To divide a mixed number by a whole number

To divide a mixed number by a whole number, follow these steps:

Step 1: Turn the mixed number into an improper fraction.

Step 2: Turn the whole number into a fraction.

Step 3: Change the division problem into multiplication by the reciprocal.

To divide a mixed number by a fraction

To divide a mixed number by a fraction, turn the mixed number into an improper fraction. Next, multiply by the reciprocal of the divisor.

To divide a fraction by a mixed number

To divide a fraction by a mixed number, turn the mixed number into an improper fraction. Next, multiply by the reciprocal of the divisor.

To divide a mixed number by a mixed number

To divide a mixed number by a mixed number, turn both mixed numbers into improper fractions. Next, multiply by the reciprocal of the divisor.

To solve division applications

Division is used to take a larger quantity and divide it into an equal number of smaller parts.

The following key words may indicate the need to divide: *per, average,* and *how much is each one.*

For example, if $20 is being evenly split among 5 children, then $20 would be divided by 5 to get $4 as an answer. Thus, each child would get $4. To verify that this is correct, consider the reverse: if each child put his or her $4 together with the others, then they would have $20. ($4 \times 5 = $20.)

CUMULATIVE TEST

(The answers are on pages 168–172.)

Identify the following as proper fraction, improper fraction, or mixed number.

1) $\frac{7}{2}$

2) $2\frac{3}{5}$

3) $\frac{9}{16}$

4) $\frac{4}{3}$

Reduce these fractions to their lowest terms.

5) $\frac{6}{12}$

6) $\frac{8}{10}$

7) $\frac{9}{21}$

8) $\frac{35}{40}$

Change these improper fractions to either whole numbers or mixed numbers.

9) $\frac{9}{4}$

10) $\frac{12}{5}$

11) $\frac{24}{8}$

12) $\frac{11}{3}$

Change these whole numbers and mixed numbers to improper fractions.

13) $2\frac{3}{4}$ 14) 12 15) $4\frac{3}{5}$ 16) $1\frac{2}{3}$

17) What is the least common multiple of 2, 3, and 4?

Raise each fraction to its equivalent higher term by supplying the missing numerator.

18) $\frac{3}{4} = \frac{}{12}$ 19) $\frac{4}{5} = \frac{}{15}$ 20) $\frac{2}{3} = \frac{}{18}$

Add these fractions. Change fractions to like denominators when necessary. If the answer is an improper fraction, convert it to a mixed number. Reduce if possible.

21) $\begin{array}{r} \frac{3}{7} \\ +\frac{2}{7} \\ \hline \end{array}$ 22) $\begin{array}{r} \frac{3}{5} \\ +\frac{2}{5} \\ \hline \end{array}$ 23) $\begin{array}{r} \frac{3}{8} \\ +\frac{1}{4} \\ \hline \end{array}$

24) $2\frac{1}{2}$

$+3\frac{3}{4}$

25) $1\frac{1}{8}$

$+3\frac{5}{8}$

26) $2\frac{1}{3}$

$+3\frac{3}{4}$

Subtract these problems. Borrow when necessary. Reduce your final answer.

27) $\frac{9}{16}$

$-\frac{3}{16}$

28) $5\frac{4}{5}$

$-2\frac{3}{5}$

29) $\frac{7}{8}$

$-\frac{1}{4}$

30) $7\frac{5}{6}$

$-3\frac{2}{3}$

31) 1

$-\frac{3}{8}$

32) 6

$-\frac{4}{5}$

33) $4\frac{1}{3}$

$-1\frac{2}{3}$

34) $9\frac{1}{4}$

$-4\frac{5}{8}$

35) $7\frac{1}{4}$

$-2\frac{5}{6}$

Multiply these fractions. Reduce the answer if possible.

36) $\frac{1}{3} \times \frac{2}{5}$

37) $\frac{3}{5} \times \frac{2}{5}$

38) $\frac{1}{2} \times \frac{1}{3} \times \frac{1}{4}$

39) $\frac{2}{3} \times \frac{3}{4}$

40) $\frac{5}{8} \times \frac{2}{5}$

41) $\frac{4}{5} \times \frac{2}{3} \times \frac{15}{16}$

42) $4 \times \frac{1}{2}$

43) $\frac{2}{3} \times 9$

44) $4 \times \frac{1}{3} \times \frac{9}{16}$

45) $1\frac{1}{4} \times 2\frac{1}{2}$

46) $4\frac{1}{6} \times 2\frac{2}{5}$

What are the reciprocals of these numbers?

47) $\frac{2}{5}$

48) $\frac{9}{16}$

49) 4

50) $\frac{1}{2}$

Solve these division problems by multiplying by the reciprocal. Turn improper fractions into mixed numbers and reduce if necessary.

51) $\frac{1}{3} \div \frac{2}{3}$

52) $\frac{3}{4} \div \frac{3}{8}$

53) $\frac{5}{8} \div 10$

54) $6 \div \frac{3}{16}$

55) $1\frac{1}{8} \div 6$

56) $2\frac{2}{3} \div \frac{4}{9}$

57) $\frac{3}{8} \div 2\frac{1}{4}$

58) $2\frac{1}{3} \div 4\frac{2}{3}$

59) A patient's fluid intake is being carefully monitored. The patient drank $4\frac{3}{4}$ oz of juice, $5\frac{1}{2}$ oz of coffee, and $6\frac{1}{4}$ oz of water. How much fluid did the patient drink?

60) A patient drank $6\frac{3}{4}$ oz out of an 8-oz glass of water. How much water was left in the glass?

61) A bottle contains 24 oz of a liquid pain reliever. If a child's dose is $\frac{3}{4}$ oz, how many doses are there in the bottle?

62) A bottle contains $10\frac{1}{2}$ oz of water. How many oz of water are there in 8 bottles?

63) A $33\frac{3}{4}$ oz supply of iced tea was divided evenly among 5 residents in an assisted living facility. How much iced tea did each resident receive?

64) A patient drank $\frac{1}{2}$ of a 16-oz bottle of water. How many oz of water did the patient drink?

65) Resident A is given $1\frac{1}{2}$ tablets of pain reliever 3 times a day for 5 days. Resident B is given $1\frac{1}{2}$ tablets of pain reliever 2 times a day for 7 days. Which resident received more tablets of medication?

ANSWERS TO CUMULATIVE TEST

(The test is on pages 161–167.)

1) $\frac{7}{2}$ is an improper fraction.

2) $2\frac{3}{5}$ is a mixed number.

3) $\frac{9}{16}$ is a proper fraction.

4) $\frac{4}{3}$ is an improper fraction.

5) $\frac{6}{12} = \frac{6 \div 6}{12 \div 6} = \frac{1}{2}$

6) $\frac{8}{10} = \frac{8 \div 2}{10 \div 2} = \frac{4}{5}$

7) $\frac{9}{21} = \frac{9 \div 3}{21 \div 3} = \frac{3}{7}$

8) $\frac{35}{40} = \frac{35 \div 5}{40 \div 5} = \frac{7}{8}$

9) $\frac{9}{4} = 2\frac{1}{4}$

10) $\frac{12}{5} = 2\frac{2}{5}$

11) $\frac{24}{8} = 3$

12) $\frac{11}{3} = 3\frac{2}{3}$

13) $2\frac{3}{4} = \frac{11}{4}$

14) $12 = \frac{12}{1}$

15) $4\frac{3}{5} = \frac{23}{5}$

16) $1\frac{2}{3} = \frac{5}{3}$

17) The least common multiple of 2, 3, and 4 is 12.
Multiples of 4: 4, 8, <u>12</u>, 16 …
Multiples of 3: 3, 6, 9, <u>12</u>, 15 …
Multiples of 2: 2, 4, 6, 8, 10, <u>12</u>, 14 …

18) $\frac{3}{4} = \frac{9}{12}$

19) $\frac{4}{5} = \frac{12}{15}$

20) $\frac{2}{3} = \frac{12}{18}$

21) $\begin{array}{r} \frac{3}{7} \\ +\frac{2}{7} \\ \hline \frac{5}{7} \end{array}$

22) $\begin{array}{r} \frac{3}{5} \\ +\frac{2}{5} \\ \hline \frac{5}{5}=1 \end{array}$

23) $\begin{array}{r} \frac{3}{8}=\frac{3}{8} \\ +\frac{1}{4}=\frac{2}{8} \\ \hline \frac{5}{8} \end{array}$

24) $\begin{aligned} 2\tfrac{1}{2} &= 2\tfrac{2}{4} \\ +3\tfrac{3}{4} &= 3\tfrac{3}{4} \\ \hline 5\tfrac{5}{4} &= 6\tfrac{1}{4} \end{aligned}$

25) $\begin{aligned} 1\tfrac{1}{8} \\ +3\tfrac{5}{8} \\ \hline 4\tfrac{6}{8} = 4\tfrac{3}{4} \end{aligned}$

26) $\begin{aligned} 2\tfrac{1}{3} &= 2\tfrac{4}{12} \\ +3\tfrac{3}{4} &= 3\tfrac{9}{12} \\ \hline 5\tfrac{13}{12} &= 6\tfrac{1}{12} \end{aligned}$

27) $\begin{aligned} \tfrac{9}{16} \\ -\tfrac{3}{16} \\ \hline \tfrac{6}{16} = \tfrac{3}{8} \end{aligned}$

28) $\begin{aligned} 5\tfrac{4}{5} \\ -2\tfrac{3}{5} \\ \hline 3\tfrac{1}{5} \end{aligned}$

29) $\begin{aligned} \tfrac{7}{8} &= \tfrac{7}{8} \\ -\tfrac{1}{4} &= \tfrac{2}{8} \\ \hline &\;\; \tfrac{5}{8} \end{aligned}$

30) $\begin{aligned} 7\tfrac{5}{6} &= 7\tfrac{5}{6} \\ -3\tfrac{2}{3} &= 3\tfrac{4}{6} \\ \hline 4\tfrac{1}{6} \end{aligned}$

31) $\begin{aligned} 1\;\; &= \tfrac{8}{8} \\ -\tfrac{3}{8} &= \tfrac{3}{8} \\ \hline &\;\; \tfrac{5}{8} \end{aligned}$

32) $\begin{aligned} 6\;\; &= 5\tfrac{5}{5} \\ -\tfrac{4}{5} &= \;\; \tfrac{4}{5} \\ \hline &\;\; 5\tfrac{1}{5} \end{aligned}$

33) $\begin{aligned} 4\tfrac{1}{3} &= 3\tfrac{4}{3} \\ -1\tfrac{2}{3} &= 1\tfrac{2}{3} \\ \hline 2\tfrac{2}{3} \end{aligned}$

34) $\begin{aligned} 9\tfrac{1}{4} &= 9\tfrac{2}{8} = 8\tfrac{10}{8} \\ -4\tfrac{5}{8} &= 4\tfrac{5}{8} = \;\; 4\tfrac{5}{8} \\ \hline 4\tfrac{5}{8} \end{aligned}$

35) $\begin{aligned} 7\tfrac{1}{4} &= 7\tfrac{3}{12} = 6\tfrac{15}{12} \\ -2\tfrac{5}{6} &= 2\tfrac{10}{12} = 2\tfrac{10}{12} \\ \hline 4\tfrac{5}{12} \end{aligned}$

36) $\dfrac{1}{3} \times \dfrac{2}{5} = \dfrac{1 \times 2}{3 \times 5} = \dfrac{2}{15}$

37) $\dfrac{3}{5} \times \dfrac{2}{5} = \dfrac{3 \times 2}{5 \times 5} = \dfrac{6}{25}$

38) $\dfrac{1}{2} \times \dfrac{1}{3} \times \dfrac{1}{4} = \dfrac{1 \times 1 \times 1}{2 \times 3 \times 4} = \dfrac{1}{24}$

39) $\dfrac{\overset{1}{\cancel{2}}}{\underset{1}{\cancel{3}}} \times \dfrac{\overset{1}{\cancel{3}}}{\underset{2}{\cancel{4}}} = \dfrac{1 \times 1}{1 \times 2} = \dfrac{1}{2}$

40) $\dfrac{5}{8} \times \dfrac{2}{5} = \dfrac{\overset{1}{\cancel{5}}}{\underset{4}{\cancel{8}}} \times \dfrac{\overset{1}{\cancel{2}}}{\underset{1}{\cancel{5}}} = \dfrac{1 \times 1}{4 \times 1} = \dfrac{1}{4}$

41) $\dfrac{4}{5} \times \dfrac{2}{3} \times \dfrac{15}{16} = \dfrac{\overset{1}{\cancel{4}}}{\underset{1}{\cancel{5}}} \times \dfrac{\overset{1}{\cancel{2}}}{\underset{1}{\cancel{3}}} \times \dfrac{\overset{\overset{1}{\cancel{3}}}{\cancel{15}}}{\underset{\underset{2}{\cancel{4}}}{\cancel{16}}} = \dfrac{1 \times 1 \times 1}{1 \times 1 \times 2} = \dfrac{1}{2}$

42) $4 \times \frac{1}{2} = \frac{\overset{2}{\cancel{4}}}{1} \times \frac{1}{\underset{1}{\cancel{2}}} \times \frac{2 \times 1}{1 \times 1} = \frac{2}{1} = 2$

43) $\frac{2}{3} \times 9 = \frac{2}{\cancel{3}} \times \frac{\overset{3}{\cancel{9}}}{1} = \frac{2 \times 3}{1 \times 1} = \frac{6}{1} = 6$

44) $4 \times \frac{1}{3} \times \frac{9}{16} = \frac{\overset{1}{\cancel{4}}}{1} \times \frac{1}{\underset{1}{\cancel{3}}} \times \frac{\overset{3}{\cancel{9}}}{\underset{4}{\cancel{16}}} = \frac{1 \times 1 \times 3}{1 \times 1 \times 4} = \frac{3}{4}$

45) $1\frac{1}{4} \times 2\frac{1}{2} = \frac{5}{4} \times \frac{5}{2} = \frac{5 \times 5}{4 \times 2} = \frac{25}{8} = 3\frac{1}{8}$

46) $4\frac{1}{6} \times 2\frac{2}{5} = \frac{25}{6} \times \frac{12}{5} = \frac{\overset{5}{\cancel{25}}}{\underset{1}{\cancel{6}}} \times \frac{\overset{2}{\cancel{12}}}{\underset{1}{\cancel{5}}} = \frac{5 \times 2}{1 \times 1} = \frac{10}{1} = 10$

47) The reciprocal of $\frac{2}{5}$ is $\frac{5}{2}$

48) The reciprocal of $\frac{9}{16}$ is $\frac{16}{9}$

49) The reciprocal of 4 is $\frac{1}{4}$

50) The reciprocal of $\frac{1}{2}$ is 2

51) $\frac{1}{3} \div \frac{2}{3} = \frac{1}{3} \times \frac{3}{2} = \frac{1}{\cancel{3}} \times \frac{\overset{1}{\cancel{3}}}{2} = \frac{1 \times 1}{1 \times 2} = \frac{1}{2}$

52) $\frac{3}{4} \div \frac{3}{8} = \frac{3}{4} \times \frac{8}{3} = \frac{\overset{1}{\cancel{3}}}{\underset{1}{\cancel{4}}} \times \frac{\overset{2}{\cancel{8}}}{\underset{1}{\cancel{3}}} = \frac{1 \times 2}{1 \times 1} = \frac{2}{1} = 2$

53) $\frac{5}{8} \div 10 = \frac{5}{8} \times \frac{1}{10} = \frac{\overset{1}{\cancel{5}}}{8} \times \frac{1}{\underset{2}{\cancel{10}}} = \frac{1 \times 1}{8 \times 2} = \frac{1}{16}$

54) $6 \div \frac{3}{16} = \frac{6}{1} \times \frac{16}{3} = \frac{\overset{2}{\cancel{6}}}{1} \times \frac{16}{\underset{1}{\cancel{3}}} = \frac{2 \times 16}{1 \times 1} = \frac{32}{1} = 32$

55) $1\frac{1}{8} \div 6 = \frac{9}{8} \times \frac{1}{6} = \frac{\overset{3}{\cancel{9}}}{8} \times \frac{1}{\underset{2}{\cancel{6}}} = \frac{3 \times 1}{8 \times 2} = \frac{3}{16}$

56) $2\frac{2}{3} \div \frac{4}{9} = \frac{8}{3} \times \frac{9}{4} = \frac{\overset{2}{\cancel{8}}}{\underset{1}{\cancel{3}}} \times \frac{\overset{3}{\cancel{9}}}{\underset{1}{\cancel{4}}} = \frac{2 \times 3}{1 \times 1} = \frac{6}{1} = 6$

57) $\frac{3}{8} \div 2\frac{1}{4} = \frac{3}{8} \div \frac{9}{4} = \frac{3}{8} \times \frac{4}{9} = \frac{\overset{1}{\cancel{3}}}{\underset{2}{\cancel{8}}} \times \frac{\overset{1}{\cancel{4}}}{\underset{3}{\cancel{9}}} = \frac{1 \times 1}{2 \times 3} = \frac{1}{6}$

58) $2\frac{1}{3} \div 4\frac{2}{3} = \frac{7}{3} \div \frac{14}{3} = \frac{7}{3} \times \frac{3}{14} = \frac{\overset{1}{\cancel{7}}}{\underset{1}{\cancel{3}}} \times \frac{\overset{1}{\cancel{3}}}{\underset{2}{\cancel{14}}} = \frac{1 \times 1}{1 \times 2} = \frac{1}{2}$

59)

$$\begin{array}{r} 4\frac{3}{4} = 4\frac{3}{4} \\ 5\frac{1}{2} = 5\frac{2}{4} \\ +6\frac{1}{4} = 6\frac{1}{4} \\ \hline 15\frac{6}{4} = 16\frac{2}{4} = 16\frac{1}{2} \end{array}$$

Add the amounts of fluid to get the total amount of fluid the patient drank. The patient drank $16\frac{1}{2}$ oz of fluid.

60)

$$\begin{array}{r} 8 = 7\frac{4}{4} \\ -6\frac{3}{4} = 6\frac{3}{4} \\ \hline 1\frac{1}{4} \end{array}$$

Subtract how many oz of water the patient drank from the total number of oz in the glass to find how much water was left. There were $1\frac{1}{4}$ oz of water left in the glass.

61) Divide the total number of oz in the bottle by the amount of one child's dose to find how many doses there are in the bottle. There are 32 of the $\frac{3}{4}$ oz doses in the bottle.

$$24 \div \frac{3}{4} = \frac{24}{1} \times \frac{4}{3} = \frac{\overset{8}{\cancel{24}}}{1} \times \frac{4}{\underset{1}{\cancel{3}}} = \frac{8 \times 4}{1 \times 1} = \frac{32}{1} = 32$$

62) Multiply the number of oz in one bottle by the number of bottles to find how many oz are in all the bottles. There are 84 oz of water in the 8 bottles.

$$10\frac{1}{2} \times 8 = \frac{21}{2} \times \frac{8}{1} = \frac{21}{\underset{1}{\cancel{2}}} \times \frac{\overset{4}{\cancel{8}}}{1} = \frac{21 \times 4}{1 \times 1} = \frac{84}{1} = 84$$

63) Divide the supply of iced tea by the 5 residents to find how much iced tea each resident received. Each resident received $6\frac{3}{4}$ oz of iced tea.

$$33\frac{3}{4} \div 5 = \frac{135}{4} \div \frac{5}{1} = \frac{135}{4} \times \frac{1}{5} = \frac{\overset{27}{\cancel{135}}}{4} \times \frac{1}{\underset{1}{\cancel{5}}} = \frac{27 \times 1}{4 \times 1} = \frac{27}{4} = 6\frac{3}{4}$$

64) Multiply the 16-oz bottle of water by $\frac{1}{2}$ to find how many oz of water the patient drank. The patient drank 8 oz.

$$16 \times \frac{1}{2} = \frac{\overset{8}{\cancel{16}}}{1} \times \frac{1}{\underset{1}{\cancel{2}}} = \frac{8 \times 1}{1 \times 1} = \frac{8}{1} = 8$$

65) Multiply <u>the number of tablets in the dose</u> times <u>how many times a day a dose was given</u> times <u>the number of days</u> to find how many tablets of medication each resident was given. Then, compare the answers to see which resident received more tablets. Resident A received more tablets.

Resident A: $1\frac{1}{2} \times 3 \times 5 = \frac{3}{2} \times \frac{3}{1} \times \frac{5}{1} = \frac{3 \times 3 \times 5}{2 \times 1 \times 1} = \frac{45}{2} = 22\frac{1}{2}$

Resident B: $1\frac{1}{2} \times 2 \times 7 = \frac{3}{2} \times \frac{\overset{1}{\cancel{2}}}{1} \times \frac{7}{1} = \frac{3 \times 1 \times 7}{1 \times 1 \times 1} = \frac{21}{1} = 21$

INDEX